PHARMACOLOGY – RESEARCH, SAFETY TESTING
AND REGULATION

DEVELOPMENT OF NEW MDR-TUBERCULOSIS DRUGS

PHARMACOLOGY – RESEARCH, SAFETY TESTING AND REGULATION

Additional books in this series can be found on Nova's website under the Series tab.

Additional E-books in this series can be found on Nova's website under the E-books tab.

PHARMACOLOGY – RESEARCH, SAFETY TESTING
AND REGULATION

DEVELOPMENT OF NEW MDR-TUBERCULOSIS DRUGS

JARMILA VINŠOVÁ

AND

MARTIN KRÁTKÝ

Nova Biomedical
Nova Science Publishers, Inc.
New York

LIBRARY OF CONGRESS CATALOGING-IN-PUBLICATION DATA
Vinova, Jarmila.
 Development of new MDR-tuberculosis drugs / Jarmila Vinova and Martin Kratk}.
 p. ; cm.
 Includes bibliographical references and index.
 ISBN 978-1-61668-233-0 (softcover)
 1. Antitubercular agents. 2. Multidrug-resistant
tuberculosis--Chemotherapy. I. Kratk}, Martin, 1960- II. Title.
 [DNLM: 1. Tuberculosis, Multidrug-Resistant--drug therapy. 2. Drug
Discovery. 3. Drug Resistance, Multiple--drug effects. WF 360 V788d 2010]
 RM409.V56 2010
 615.5'8--dc22
 2010002978

Published by Nova Science Publishers, Inc. ; New York

CONTENTS

PREFACE

The aim of this review is to outline the recent advances in the development of new multidrug-resistant tuberculosis (MDR-TB) drugs. The emergence of resistance to antituberculosis drugs, particularly of MDR-TB and newly XDR-TB, has become a major public health problem. The current treatment regiment has several disadvantages, *i.e.* long treatment period (DOTS takes minimum 6 months) during which tubercle bacilli mutant becomes resistant to one or more drugs; side effects of the used drugs; co-infection of HIV/AIDS. The emergence of MDR-TB has made many currently available anti-TB drugs ineffective. Sleeping latent forms of mutant bacilli resistant against common anti-TB drugs are the risk of epidemic for the new generation. Therefore, there is an urgent need to identify new drug targets and to find novel chemical structures active especially against MDR-TB.

In general, drug resistance mechanisms in *Mycobacterium tuberculosis* are caused by mutations in chromosomal genes. It includes target modifications, barrier mechanism, inactivation or activation of enzymes, mutation in the genes as *inhA*, *rpoB*, *rpsL*, *rrs*, *emrB* and *gyrA*, responsible for INH, RIF, STM, EMB and quinolone resistances. Some novel targets as an essential cell division protein (FtsZ), ATP-synthase target, isocitrate lyase, targeting P450 enzymes etc. are presented. The research of novel MDR potential drugs follows six main strategies: a) structure modification of known compounds (INH, RIF, PZA, ETH, EMB, quinolones); b) new leads with novel mechanism of the action (linezolid, TMC207, PA-824, OPC-67683, BM212, SQ109, FAS20013, LL-3858); c) novel drug targets, *i.e.* cell wall biosynthesis (mycolic acid synthesis, protein synthesis, arabinogalactan and peptidoglycan biosynthesis inhibitors) or other novel targets like enzymes; d) investigation of "non-antituberculous" drugs; e) testing of newly prepared synthetic compounds without known mechanism of the action; f) screening of natural products, determination and isolation of active compounds.

INTRODUCTION

The increasing emergence of drug-resistant tuberculosis, especially multidrug-resistant tuberculosis (MDR-TB) and the most recent extremely drug-resistant tuberculosis (XDR-TB) is alarming [1,2,3]. It is estimated that one third of the world's population (about 2 billion people) are currently infected with *Mycobacterium tuberculosis* (*M. tbc.*), and each year 8 to 9 million new cases develop and 1.6 million die as a result. Every year almost 500,000 people are infected with MDR-TB and there are an estimated 40,000 new cases of extensively drug-resistant TB (XDR-TB) annually [4,5]. A proportion of MDR-TB among newly-diagnosed tuberculosis is presented in Figure 1.

In the early 1990s, a multidrug-resistant *Mycobacterium tuberculosis* strain was identified and defined as resistant to at least the two most effective anti-TB drug: isoniazid (INH) and rifampicin (RIF; rifampin is a synonymous term); it may include resistance to more antituberculotics. Approximately 50% of the MDR-TB cases are resistant to the four of the first-line drugs (Table 1) – INH, RIF, pyrazinamide (PZA), and ethambutol (EMB) [6]. Directly-observed therapy short-course (DOTS) requires a daily use of these four drugs for two months (the intensive phase leading to the destruction of bacteria in all growth stages) and two drugs (INH and RIF) daily for four months (the continuation phase when any residual dormant bacilli are eliminated) [7]. Treating the MDR-TB patient requires a minimum of 18-24 months.

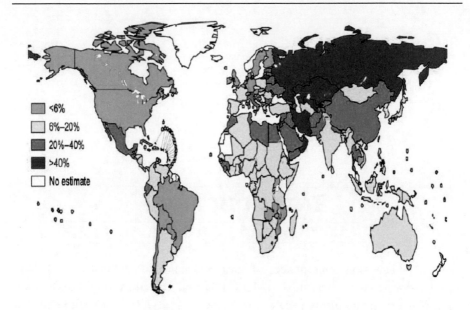

Figure 1. Percentage of MDR-TB among new TB cases in 2006 (this picture was taken from [6]).

The MDR phenotype of *M. tbc.* is not caused by a single pleiotropic mutation, but it is caused by the sequential accumulation of mutations involving different genes which induce resistance to a single type of drugs, due to an inadequate treatment or a bad adherence to the treatment [8].

Extensively or extremely drug-resistant tuberculosis (XDR-TB) was defined in 2006 as a resistance to any fluoroquinolone (FQ) and to at least one of the three injectable drugs, capreomycin, kanamycin, or amikacin, which are called second-line TB drugs, in addition to MDR-TB (resistance at least to rifampicin and isoniazid, the two most powerful antituberculotics of the first-line) [9,10]. XDR-TB is very often untreatable. Other lethal co-infection with immunocompromise patients (HIV) presents a serious challenge for the research to find a new type of drug or prodrug that is active against MDR-TB by a different mechanism of the action. Over the past 40 years, no new drug classes except rifabutin and rifapentin have been introduced to the treatment of tuberculosis. Therefore, the research on the mechanism of the action of existing drugs and novel drug targets and types of effective molecules is important.

**Table 1. Classification of drugs used for the treatment of tuberculosis
(freely according to [12])**

Group 1: First-line oral antituberculotics		
isoniazid	rifampicin	pyrazinamide
rifabutin	ethambutol	
Group 2: Injectable antituberculotics		
amikacin	kanamycin	(viomycin)
capreomycin	streptomycin	
Group 3: Fluoroquinolones		
ofloxacin	moxifloxacin	
levofloxacin	(gatifloxacin)	
Group 4: Second-line oral antituberculotics		
cycloserine	prothionamide	p-aminosalicylic acid
ethionamide	terizidone	
Group 5: Drugs with unclear role in DR-TB treatment		
amoxicillin/clavulanate		clarithromycin
imipenem/cilastatin		clofazimine
high-dose isoniazid		linezolid
thioacetazone		

A general drug resistance mechanism consists of the target modification, over-expression, and the highly hydrophobic mycobacterial cell envelope barrier mechanism. The presence of drug inactivating enzymes, or decreased levels of activating enzymes, may also contribute to the drug-resistance. *M. tbc.* target modifications are mutations in *inhA*, *rpoB*, *rpsL* or *rrs*, *emrB* and *gyrA*, responsible for INH, RIF, streptomycin (STM), ethionamide (ETH), and quinolone resistances. In general, the drug resistance in *M. tbc.* is caused by mutations in chromosomal genes.

The long-current drug regiments, the emergency of drug resistant strains, and HIV co-infection have resulted in the resurgence in research efforts to address the urgent need for new antituberculosis drugs.

The drugs have been divided in the above table into five groups depending on decreasing efficacy and tolerability. In the first group, first-line oral antituberculotics are the most potent and well-tolerated drugs. Kanamycin or amikacin are preferred as the first choice of injectable agents in group 2 because of the high rate of streptomycin resistance and because they have less ototoxicity than streptomycin. Viomycin could be considered as belonging to these named drugs. In group 3, ciprofloxacin is missing because it is no longer recommended to treat drug-susceptible or drug-resistant TB due to its weak efficacy in comparison with other quinolones; on the other side, gatifloxacin showed the same *in vitro* activity-like moxifloxacin. Group 4 is called classical second-line oral antituberculotics. Group 5 drugs are not recommended by WHO for a routine use in the drug-resistant tuberculosis treatment because their contribution to the efficacy of multidrug regiments is unclear. They have demonstrated some activity *in vitro* or in animal models, but there is little or no evidence of their efficacy in humans. Thioacetazone has a known activity against TB, but its role in the MDR-TB treatment is not well established, therefore it is included in group 5, too [12].

The treatment of MDR tuberculosis is quite challenging. There are three main goals of the development:

1) New agents to shorten the duration of therapy from current 6-9 months to two months or less. Compounds with sterilizing activity are requested.
2) Development of new drugs to treat MDR-TB with novel mechanism of the action without cross-resistance.
3) Development of new drugs to improve the treatment of a latent infection.

Chapter 1

RESISTANCE TO COMMONLY USED DRUGS, MECHANISM OF THE ACTION

ISONIAZID, ETHIONAMIDE

INH is the most widely used drug. Despite its simple structure, its mode of action is one of the most complex; it interferes with nearly every metabolic pathway in *M. tbc*. INH, as well as ETH, which is structurally very similar, requires activation by *katG*-encoded catalase-peroxidase. When activated, INH-NAD, or ETH-NAD, adducts are formed and they inhibit InhA and, hence, mycolic acid biosynthesis. INH enters the cell as a prodrug [13], is activated by hemeB-containing catalase-peroxidase protein (KatG), encoded by *katG* gene in *M. tuberculosis*. Two other genes, *inhA* and *kasA*, are important in mycolic acids synthesis. The InhA, an enoyl-acyl carrier protein reductase, catalyzes NADH-specific reduction step, which is essential to the fatty acid synthesis or elongation of those long-chain fatty acids for mycolic acid synthesis. KasA, a ketoacyl-carrier protein synthase, also mediates synthesis of mycolic acids. The activation of INH may also defect DNA, proteins, and other macromolecules through the formation of reactive oxygen species. Deficient efflux (EfpA) and insufficient antagonism (AphC) of INH-derived radicals of defective antioxidative defenses may underline the unique susceptibility of *M. tbc*. to INH (Figure 2) [14]. The mechanism of activation of INH and ETH is similar but not identical; therefore, some INH-resistant strains are susceptible to ETH because of another enzyme responsible for its activation [9].

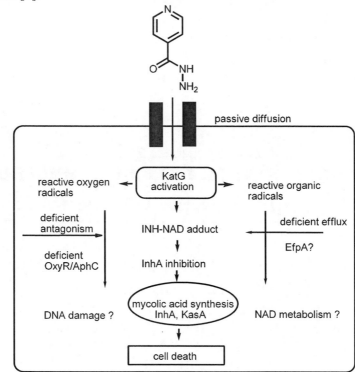

Figure 2. Model of the action of INH.

Unlike most organisms, mycobacteria have two fatty acid synthases, the fatty acid synthase I (FAS I) and FAS II systems (Figure 3). The discovery that mycobacteria had FAS I was surprising, as it is the first prokaryote shown to have FAS I, a multidomain enzyme that encodes all activities necessary for fatty acid synthesis in one large polypeptide [15].

FAS I produces saturated fatty acids in a bimodal pattern of palmitate and tetracosanoate, the acyl carrier protein (ACP)-requiring FAS II system that contains a series of independent enzymes, including InhA and KasA/B responsible for the biosynthesis of mycolic acid by the elongation of the FAS I products [16]. FAS I carries on the synthesis of C_{16} to $C_{24/26}$ which are substrates for the synthesis of mycolic acids by FAS II. Putative targets for the activated INH are underlined.

INH- and ETH-resistance involves inactivation of activators (KatG or EthA), the target over expression or the target alteration and the presence of NADH/NAD levels modulators inside the cells.

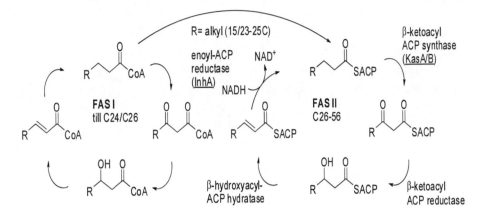

Figure 3. FAS I and II systems.

The main targets are mutations in the *katG* and *inhA* genes. A deletion or a mutation of the *katG* gene leads to the high level of INH-resistance and renders the bacteria catalase negative [17]. S315T mutation is the most common and occurs in about 50-93% [18]. It was found that S94A mutation was responsible for INH resistance and co-resistance to ETH. Amino acid replacements in the NADH binding site of InhA apparently result in INH resistance by preventing the inhibition of mycolic acid biosynthesis. Mutations in the KatG or InhA do not account for all INH-resistant strains since 15-25% of INH-resistant clinical isolates have both wild-type *katG* and *inhA* genes. Mutations in the KatG account for approximately two-thirds of INH-resistance. The basis of INH-resistance was determined by cell-free mycolic acid synthesis assays. The mutation of the InhA enzyme that causes specific reduction of 2-*trans*-enoyl acyl carrier protein, an essential step in fatty acid elongation, catalyzed by NADH is one possible source of resistance.

KatG of *M. tuberculosis* is a catalase-peroxidase, which is composed of 735 amino acids and its molecular weight is 80 kDa [19]. Twenty-five different polymorphisms of KatG have been described. Most of the frequently identified amino acid substitutions identified in clinical isolates 463 Arg → Leu [20], 315 Ser → Thr [21] are believed to be associated with INH-resistance.

Telenti et al. [22] analyzed *M. tuberculosis* isolates by PCR and found that the mutation frequencies were as follows for INH-resistant strains: KatG (36.8%), *inhA* (31.6%), KatG-*inhA* (2.6%), *ahpC* (13.2%), and KatG-*ahpC* (2.6%).

There are other genes, whose mutations are responsible for INH resistance, e.g. *kasA*, but a frequency of its occurrence is low and its association with the resistance was not investigated very well [9].

The mutation rate leading to INH-resistance is 100 times higher than that responsible for rifampicin-resistance [23].

RIFAMPICIN

RIF is not specific for *M. tbc.*; it has a bactericidal broad spectrum against the growing and stationary phase bacilli with a mechanism of the action as an inhibitor of RNA synthesis by binding to the β-subunit of bacterial RNA polymerase in bacterial cells. The mechanism of the resistance to RIF is caused by a mutation in the *rpoB* gene encoding β-subunit of the RNA polymerase and is the same as in other bacteria. Mutations in a defined 81-bp region of *rpoB* (rifampicin-resistance determining region) are found in the majority of RIF-resistant *M. tbc.* isolates [9,20]. These mutations result in conformational changes causing the low affinity for RIF, and they are clustered in three regions in the central region of the β-subunit gene – amino acids 512-534, 563-574, and 687. Their mutations are usually linked to the high-level of resistance and crossed with the resistance to other rifamycins. Mutations in codons 511, 516, 518, 522, 529, and 533 have been associated with the low-level resistance to RIF and the susceptibility with other rifamycins [9].

PYRAZINAMIDE

PZA plays an important role in shortening the therapy because it kills non-growing persisting tubercle bacilli in an acidic pH in the lesion that are not killed by other TB drugs [24,25]. It can show bactericidal or bacteriostatic activity depending on metabolic status of tubercle bacilli, pH, oxygen tension, and drug concentration. PZA is a prodrug that has to be converted to the active form pyrazinoic acid (POA) by pyrazinamidase (PZase; nicotinamidase enzyme) encoded by the *pncA* gene [26]. POA is formed in the neutral cytoplasmic environment as the anion. The anion is acidified, then enters the cell, accumulates there, and kills the bacterial cell. PZA resistance is associated with the loss of pyrazinamidase (PZase) and nicotinamidase activity. The major mechanisms of the PZA-resistance are the *pncA* mutations [27,28]. It exists in a wide range of alterations of *pnc*A gene in PZA-resistant strains, typically in the 82 bp (promotor region) or 630 bp (open reading frame), but some resistant strains do not show any alteration in the promotor or coding region of this gene. It is supposed that this resistance could be caused due to the mutation of an unknown regulatory gene [9,26].

ETHAMBUTOL

EMB is a synthetic compound with a structural similarity to D-arabinose with *S,S* absolute configuration that is essential for a bacteriostatic property. Its effect includes the inhibition of RNA metabolism, phospholipids synthesis, transfer of mycolic acids to cell wall-linked arabinogalactan, spermidine synthesis, and early steps of glucose conversion into the constituent monosaccharides such as arabinogalactan and arabinomannan. EMB could conceivably behave as an arabinose mimetic [14].

Arabinogalactane biosynthesis is dependent on the activity of the *emb*CAB gene cluster [29], which encodes the arabinotransferase that mediates the polymerization of arabinose into arabinan. These enzymes are considered as the targets for EMB. Most of EMB-resistant strains were associated with a single gene mutation in *embB,* whereas the majority of these mutations respond to the replacement of amino acid at positions 306 (wild-type phenotype Met is replaced by Ile, Leu, or Val), 406 (Gly was altered to Ala, Asp, Cys, or Ser), and others. These mutations led to the increase of EMB MIC in the different rates. Polymorphisms in *emb*A and *emb*C genes are partly responsible for EMB-resistance, too. Some of the mutations in the *embC-embA* region affect a putative TATA box. Resistance-associated mutations were also identified in several genes, e.g. *iniA* or *Rv3124* [9,30].

Table 2. Mechanisms of the action of conventional TB drugs and resistance in *M. tbc.* [35]

Drug	MIC (µg/mL)	Gene(s) involved in resistance	Gene function	Role	Mechanism of the action	Mutation (% of resistant strains)
INH	0.02-0.2	katG	catalase-peroxidase	prodrug conversion	inhibition of mycolic acid bio-synthesis and other multiple effects on DNA, lipids, carbo-hydrates and NAD metabolism	50-80
		inhA	enoyl-ACP reductase	drug target		15-43
		ahpC	alkylhydro-peroxide reductase	marker of resistance		10-15
ETH	2.5-10	etaA/ethA	flavin monooxyge-nase	prodrug conversion	inhibition of mycolic acid synthesis	37
		inhA		drug target		
RIF	0.5-2	rpoB	RNA polymerase	drug target	inhibition of RNA synthesis	96
PZA	16-50 (pH 5.5)	pncA	nicotinami-dase/ pyrazinami-dase	prodrug conversion	depletion of membrane energy, inhibition of FAS I	72-97
EMB	1-5	embB	arabinosyl transferase	drug target	inhibition of arabinogalactan synthesis	47-65
STM	2-8	rpsL	S12 riboso-mal protein	drug target	inhibition of protein synthesis	52-59
		rrs	16S rRNA	drug target		8-21
Amika-cin/ Kana-mycin	2-4	rrs	16S rRNA	drug target	inhibition of protein synthesis	76
Capre-omycin	1-4	rrs	16S rRNA	drug target	inhibition of protein synthesis	not available
Viomy-cin	5-20	tlyA	2'-O-methyl-transferase	drug target		not available
Quino-lones	0.5-2.5	gyrA	DNA gyrase subunit A	drug target	inhibition of DNA gyrase	75-94
		gyrB	DNA gyrase subunit B	drug target		
Drug	MIC (µg/mL)	Gene(s) involved in resistance	Gene function	Role	Mechanism of the action	Mutation (% of resistant strains)
PAS	1-8	thyA	thymidylate synthase	drug target?	inhibition of folic acid and iron metabolism?	not available

STREPTOMYCIN

STM is an aminocyclitol antibiotic that acts on ribosomes and causes a misreading of a genetic code, the inhibition of initiation of mRNA translation, and aberrant proofreading [31]. The resistance to streptomycin is based on mutations in the *rps*L gene, which encodes the ribosomal protein S12 [32]. The most common point mutation is a substitution in codon 43 Lys → Arg, less common is a substitution Lys → Thr [9]. Additional mutations conferring streptomycin resistance have been found in 16s rRNA gene *rrs*, and these mutations affect the conserved regions around nucleotides 530 and 912 [33]. Both mutations result in high or intermediate levels of STM-resistance, but there are some STM-resistant strains without *rps*L or *rrs* gene mutations. It is supposed that the low cell concentration of STM, a reason of the resistance, is caused by an activity of efflux pumps [9].

FLUOROQUINOLONES

The principle target of quinolones is DNA gyrase or topoisomerase IV enzyme, which thereby inhibits DNA replication and transcription. DNA gyrase is composed of two subunits encoded by *gyrA* and *gyrB*. Mutations in the quinolone-resistance determining regions of *gyr*A and *gyr*B have played the most important role in quinolone resistance [9,34].

Chapter 2

RESEARCH OF NOVEL MDR-POTENTIAL DRUGS

The current research involves the testing of new or transformed drugs, combinations of different drugs to shorten the therapy, a development of novel slow-release drug delivery systems that could reduce the frequency and an amount of drugs necessary during the treatment, and the research of molecular targets.

The approach includes the chemical modification of existing drugs, the identification of drug targets, structure-based drug design, and new types of structures. Besides chemotherapy and immunotherapeutic approaches such as DNA vaccines, cytokines used in the combination with chemotherapy offer a promising prospect for the treatment of TB [36].

Research trends lead to the small molecules' synthesis with the following parameters: best MIC (MIC for *M. tuberculosis* strain $H_{37}Rv$) and physico-chemical parameters as the Lipinski rule of 5, no more than 5 H-bond donors, no more than 10 H-bond acceptors, molecular weight no higher than 500 Da, clog*P* no higher than 5 (calculated octanol/water), flexibility (the number of rotable bonds in a given molecule should be kept bellow 10, and favourable toxicological profile as assessed by selectivity index (SI) [37].

1. STRUCTURE MODIFICATION OF KNOWN COMPOUNDS (INH, ETH, RIF AND RIFAMYCIN DERIVATIVES, PZA, EMB, AND QUINOLONES)

Many analogues of *isoniazid* have been synthesized and are still the subject of research [38,39,40,41]. A critical review was been published in 2006 [42]. The majority of newly-prepared isoniazid derivatives do not act on INH-resistant mycobacterial strains; hence, it could be supposed that they are prodrugs of isoniazid.

One of the successful modifications of isoniazid was its inorganic complex with a cyanoferrate moiety that inhibits mycobacterial wild-type and an isoniazid-resistant mutant 2-*trans*-enoyl-ACP (CoA) reductase. *In vitro* kinetics of inactivation of both types of enzymes by $[Fe^{II}(CN)_5(INH)]^{3-}$ (1) indicate that this process does not need activation by KatG or the presence of NADH, which are necessary for action of INH. The mechanism of the action of this complex probably involves interaction with the NADH binding site of the enzyme. As for the wild-type InhA enzyme, these results demonstrate that the inactivation of the mutant enzyme from an INH-resistant clinical isolate of *M. tuberculosis* by $[Fe^{II}(CN)_5(INH)]^{3-}$ requires no activation by KatG, no need for NADH, and probably the same site of interaction. Interestingly, this complex would probably display a better efficacy against isoniazid-resistant *M. tuberculosis* strains harboring the *inhA* structural gene mutations than wild-type InhA strains. The MIC of this compound was 0.2 µg/mL [43]. This approach of overcoming INH-resistance is based on the synthesis of a new molecule capable of promoting an inner-sphere electron transfer reaction, e.g. a redox reversible metal complex coordinated to the prodrugs like the pentacyanoferrate(II) metal centre with an isoniazid ligand with a proposing self-activation mechanism. Upon oxidation of this complex by oxygen or cellular oxidants, the thermodynamically unstable iron(III) complex would undergo a rapid intramolecular electron transfer reaction forming the $[Fe^{II}(CN)_5(isonicotinyl)]^{3-}$ intermediate species which could decay to the $[Fe^{II}(CN)_5(L)]^{3-}$ complex (L = isonicotinic acid, isonicotinamide, or isonicotinaldehyde) and bind to enoyl reductase resulting in the inhibition of mycolic acid synthesis without the interference of the KatG enzyme [44].

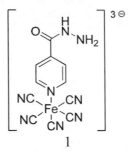

1

The peroxidase activity of mycobacterial KatG catalyzes the conversion of Mn^{2+} to Mn^{3+}. It has been shown that the yield of the isonicotinoyl-NAD adduct is about the same after oxidation of isoniazid by KatG or Mn^{3+}. In accordance with this knowledge, Mn^{3+}-pyrophosphate has been proposed to be an alternative oxidant that mimics the activity of KatG. A single INH-NAD(H) adduct in the open form with a $4S$ configuration has been detected in the active site of *M. tuberculosis* InhA by the X-ray crystallography. 1-Isonicotinoyl-2-nonanoyl hydrazine, an analogue of INH, has been demonstrated to exhibit a two-fold increase in the degree of susceptibility against *M. tuberculosis* $H_{37}Rv$. However, no data has been presented for INH-resistant strains of *M. tuberculosis* [44].

Because some pyrazole derivatives show anti-tuberculous activity, INH was incorporated in a pyrazoline moiety to form a new group, [3-(4-hydroxy-3-methylphenyl)-5-(substituted phenyl)-4,5-dihydro-1*H*-pyrazol-1-yl](pyridin-4-yl)methanones. These compounds underwent the testing *in vitro* against *M. tuberculosis* $H_{37}Rv$ and the INH-resistant clinical isolate of *M. tbc.* It was found that [5-(2-chlorophenyl)-3-(4-hydroxy-3-methylphenyl)-4,5-dihydro-1*H*-pyrazol-1-yl](pyridin-4-yl)methanone (2) was the most active agent with an MIC value of 0.26 μM, and in comparison to INH, showed 2.8- and 43.7-fold more activity against sensitive and INH-resistant *M. tbc.*, respectively. This and other compounds were further examined for toxicity in a mammalian Vero cell line at the concentration of 62.5 μg/mL with the result being non-toxic up to this concentration [45]. It is interesting that anti-mycobacterial activity against both susceptible and INH-resistant strains showed 4-[5-(substituted phenyl)-1-phenyl-4,5-dihydro-1*H*-pyrazol-3-yl]-2-methylphenol derivatives, also, which are similar to the compounds described above, and they were simplified by the replacement of the nicotinoyl group by the phenyl group. The most active of these derivatives, 4-[5-(4-fluorophenyl)-1-phenyl-4,5-dihydro-1*H*-pyrazol-3-yl]-2-methylphenol (3), showed during the testing against isoniazid-resistant *M. tuberculosis* a good anti-mycobacterial activity with a MIC value of 0.62 μg/mL [46].

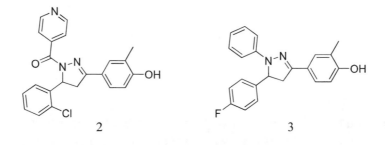

2   3

Other isoniazid derivatives with incorporated hydrazide group into heterocycle, [3-substituted-5-hydroxy-5-(trifluoro- or trichloromethyl)-4,5-dihydro-1*H*-pyrazol-1-yl](pyridin-1-yl)methanones were assessed for their *in vitro* antimicrobial activity against the INH-susceptible mycobacterial strain $H_{37}Rv$ and INH-resistant clinical isolates. Among these compounds, [5-hydroxy-5-(trifluoromethyl)-4,5-dihydro-1*H*-pyrazol-1-yl](pyridine-4-yl)-methanone (4) and {5-hydroxy-5-(trifluoromethyl)-3-[4-(trifluoromethyl)-phenyl]-4,5-dihydro-1*H*-pyrazol-1-yl}(pyridine-4-yl)methanone (5) were found to be the most active agents against susceptible *M. tbc.* and several INH-resistant strains. Whereas [3-(furan-2-yl)-5-hydroxy-5-(trifluoromethyl)-4,5-dihydro-1*H*-pyrazol-1-yl](pyridin-4-yl)methanone (6) was active against all the INH-resistant strains regardless of the genetic background at concentrations two- to four-fold of its MIC against *M. tuberculosis* $H_{37}Rv$. These compounds act as inhibitors of mycolic acid biosynthesis, in agreement with the utilization of the INH scaffold for their design. Trifluoromethyl-substituted pyrazolines were more active than their trichloromethyl analogues [47].

Other series of INH derivatives with a pyrazole ring, 2-{4-[5-(substituted phenyl)-1-isonicotinoyl-4,5-dihydro-1*H*-pyrazol-3-yl]-2-methoxyphenoxy}-acetic acids, were evaluated for their anti-mycobacterial activity *in vitro* against *M. tuberculosis* $H_{37}Rv$ and INH-resistant *M. tbc.* 2-{4-[5-(4-Hydroxyphenyl)-1-isonicotinoyl-4,5-dihydro-1*H*-pyrazol-3-yl]-2-methoxy-phenoxy}acetic acid (7) was described being the most active against *M. tuberculosis* $H_{37}Rv$ and INH-resistant *M. tuberculosis* with MIC of 0.12 μM, when compared to INH 5.6-fold more active against *M. tuberculosis* and 78-fold more active against the INH-resistant strain, respectively [48].

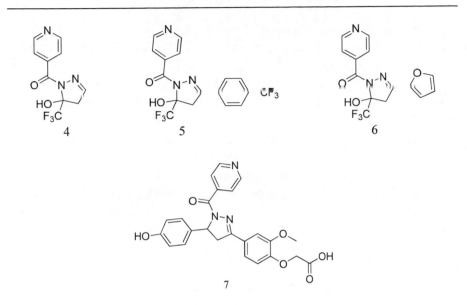

4   5   6

7

The conversion of INH to oxadiazoles produces the corresponding 2-substituted-5-(pyridin-4-yl)-1,3,4-oxadiazole derivatives characterized by their high activity against the *M. tuberculosis* strain $H_{37}Rv$. Some compounds showed an interesting activity against *Mycobacterium tuberculosis* $H_{37}Rv$ and five clinical isolates (drug-sensitive and resistant strains). 2-Pentadecyl-5-(pyridin-4-yl)-1,3,4-oxadiazole (8) was 10 times more active than isoniazid, 20 times more active than streptomycin, and 28 times more potent than ethambutol against drug-resistant strain CIBIN 112. 2-Heptadecyl-5-(pyridin-4-yl)-1,3,4-oxadiazole showed the same behavior. These structures were found to be the most potent compounds with MIC 0.35 and 0.65 μM, respectively, showing similar activity to INH (0.44 μM) against *M. tuberculosis* strain $H_{37}Rv$. Both structures bear a high lipophilic chain bonded to the 2-position of the oxadiazole moiety. This fact implies that there exists a contribution of lipophilicity, which could facilitate the entrance of these molecules through lipid-enriched bacterial cell membranes. The remaining compounds showed an activity similar to that of INH against INH-resistant strains and higher than that of INH in the sensitive clinical isolates [49].

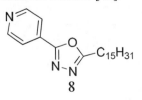

8

The series of isonicotinoylhydrazinocarbothioamides combines INH with a thioamide group, which is a part of ethionamide and prothionamide, second-line oral anti-tuberculotics. New derivatives were tested for their anti-mycobacterial activity *in vitro* against *M. tbc.* H$_{37}$Rv and INH-resistant *M. tbc.* Among the synthesized compounds, 2-isonicotinoyl-*N*-[2-(trifluoromethyl) phenyl]hydrazinecarbothioamide (9) was found to be the most potent compound with MIC of 0.58 μM against INH-susceptible and INH-resistant *M. tuberculosis*. When compared to INH, this compound was assessed to be 1.24 and 157 times more active against *M. tbc.* H$_{37}$Rv and INH-resistant strains respectively, with a selectivity index of > 218. With reference to the structure-activity relationship, substituents with strongly deactivating electron-withdrawing groups like nitro- and trifluoromethyl- groups in the phenyl ring showed an excellent anti-mycobacterial activity, while electron-donating groups (e.g. methyl and methoxy) reduced the activity. Subsequently, the named compound was tested for efficacy against *M. tbc. in vivo* at a dose of 25 mg/kg in 6-week-old female CD-1 mice. It demonstrated a decrease of bacterial load in the lungs from 7.99 colony-forming unit (CFU) to 5.61 and in spleen from 9.02 to 4.10 log protections, and, therefore, it was considered to be promising in reducing the bacterial count in lung and spleen tissues [50].

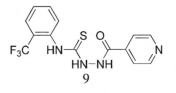

9

For the second-line anti-tubercular drugs, *ethionamide* and *prothionamide*, there is the typical pharmacophore thioamide group. Therefore, this substitution was introduced in other anti-mycobacterial potent compounds, 2-(benzylthio)benzoxazoles. Newly prepared products were evaluated, including resistant mycobacterial strains (*M. tuberculosis* 7357/98 resistant to isoniazid, rifampicin, ethambutol, streptomycin, ofloxacin, rifabutin, and ciprofloxacin; *M. tbc.* 4977/03 resistant to isoniazid, rifampicin, ethambutol, streptomycin, ofloxacin, and rifabutin, or *M. tbc.* 550/04 resistant to isoniazid, rifampicin, gentamicin, amikacin, and rifabutin. A MIC value for the most active 4-([benzoxazol-2-ylthio]methyl)benzothioamide (10) ranges for this resistant strain from 8 to 32 μM [51].

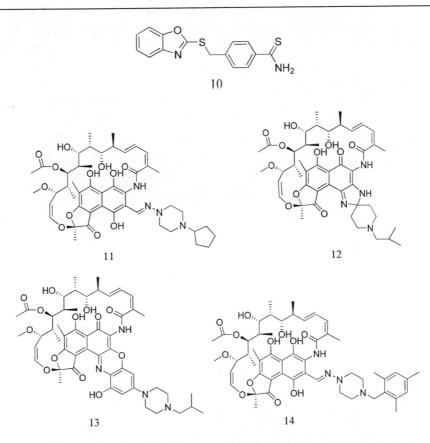

The most prominent of the new rifamycins are *rifapentin* (11), *rifabutin* (12), and *rifalazil* (13). Their long serum half-life may permit the establishment of an intermittent regimen, thus reducing the total number of dosages to be taken under DOTS supervision. Rifapentin appears to be safe, well tolerated at once weekly dosings, and is currently being evaluated in Phase III efficacy trials for the treatment of latent TB [52]. Their main problem is that their common mechanism of the action makes RIF-resistant *M. tbc.* strains cross-resistant to all rifamycins.

Rifalazil represents a new generation of ansamycins that contains a unique four-ring structure. Originally, rifalazil was developed as a therapeutic agent to replace rifampicin as a part of a multiple drug regimen in the treatment of tuberculosis. Because of its superior antimicrobial activity and high intracellular levels, rifalazil has the potential to treat indications caused by the intracellular pathogen, *Chlamydia trachomatis*, which causes non-gonococcal urethritis and cervicitis, often leading to pelvic inflammatory disease [53,54]. *CGP7040* (14) was more active than rifabutin and was superior to rifampicin towards *M. tbc*. It was found to be more stable than rifampicin [55].

Reddy et al. [56] referred in 1995 to the anti-mycobacterial activity of a rifampicin derivative 3-(4-cinnamoylpiperazinyliminomethyl)rifamycin (15), which was investigated against 20 susceptible and multidrug-resistant strains of *M. tuberculosis* and 20 *M. avium complex* strains. Its MIC for *M. tuberculosis* was significantly lower (from 2 to 8-fold) than those of RIF, and, what is important, this derivative had lower MIC (0.25-8 μg/mL) against some RIF (> 8 μg/mL) and multidrug-resistant strains of *M. tbc*.

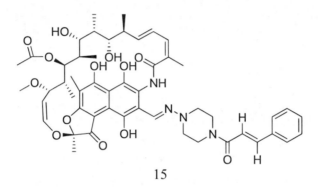

15

Clinical utility of rifabutin has been hampered due to dose-limiting toxicity. Some its analogues were synthesized and evaluated against susceptible and resistant *M. avium* and *M. tuberculosis* strains *in vitro*, against non-replicating persistent *M. tuberculosis* and subsequent *in vivo*. An important feature of the rifamycins is that they are active against both actively growing and slow metabolizing non-growing bacilli. The most active compound against *M. avium* 1581 was *N'*-acetylrifabutin (16) with MIC of 0.2 μg/mL followed by 25-deacetylrifabutin. The presence of a hydroxy group, resulting from the hydrolysis of the acetyl moiety at the ansa chain, seems to have a different impact on the *M. avium* activity depending on the presence of the furanone or furanol at C-11. The assay of activities against *M. tuberculosis* $H_{37}Rv$ showed that most of ribabutin derivatives were active against *M. tbc*. $H_{37}Rv$ at concentrations as low as 0.1 μg/mL, with the more polar *N*-oxide derivatives being an exception. The most active were rifabutin and *N'*-acetylrifabutin with MIC < 0.013 μg/mL. *N'*-Acetylrifabutinol and *N'*-(undec-10'-enoyl)-rifabutin (17) exhibiting the highest activity against MDR-

TB clinical isolates (except RIF- and INH- resistant to STM or EMB, additionally) having a MIC value of 8 and 6 µg/mL, respectively. Both the luciferase and CFU endpoints indicated that all of the rifabutin derivatives were more active against non-replicating persistent mycobacteria than RIF, especially rifabutin and N'-(undec-10´-enoyl)-rifabutin, but this derivative appears to be more cytotoxic (Vero cells) than rifabutin. Rifabutin, N'-acetylrifabutin and N'-(undec-10´-enoyl)-rifabutin were tested in a model of progressive pulmonary tuberculosis in Balb/c mice. Mice received daily these compounds in two different doses (5 or 15 mg/kg). The lower dose produced better results than the higher dose. Mice infected with susceptible strain $H_{37}Rv$ treated with N'-acetylrifabutin showed a similar CFU reduction with the rifabutin treatment, producing a threefold reduction of lung bacilli loads in comparison to the non-treated control, with non-significant lesser pneumonia, while by N'-(undec-10´-enoyl)-rifabutin treated animals showed a similar CFU and a lung surface affected by pneumonia as the mice in the control group. In animals infected with the MDR strain, the treatment with all three compounds showed similar efficacy, producing a significant, five-fold, lesser CFU than in control mice and a lesser, but not significant reduction of pneumonia [57].

A series of *pyrazinamide* Mannich basis has been synthesized and evaluated for anti-mycobacterial activity *in vitro* and *in vivo* against *Mycobacterium tuberculosis* $H_{37}Rv$. Among the synthesized compounds, 1-cyclopropyl-6-fluoro-8-methoxy-4-oxo-7-{4-[(pyrazine-2-carboxamido)-methyl]piperazin-1-yl}-1,4-dihydroquinoline-3-carboxylic acid (18) was found to be the most active compound *in vitro* with MIC of 0.39 and 0.2 µg/mL against *M. tbc.* and a multidrug-resistant strain that was resistant to isoniazid, rifampicin, pyrazinamide, and ofloxacin. This compound was > 125 times more potent than the parent drug PZA and > 7 times more potent than isoniazid (MIC = 1.56 µg/mL) against MDR-TB. The compound was tested *in vivo* and decreased the bacterial load in lung and spleen tissues at a dose of 100 mg/kg with 1.86 and 1.66 log protections, respectively. Its activity might be due to the inhibition of both mycobacterial enzymes, FAS I and DNA gyrase [58].

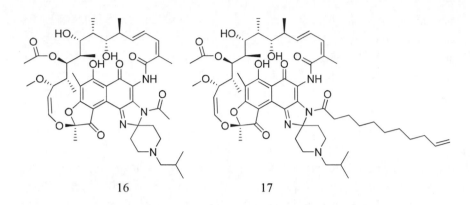

16   17

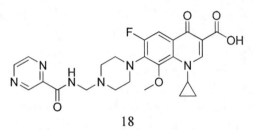

18

Many pyrazinamide derivatives with lower MIC on different tuberculous and non-tuberculous mycobacteria then pyrazinamide were synthesized, e.g. 5-chloropyrazinamide (19), propyl pyrazin-2-carboxylate (20), substituted pyrazinecarboxamides (21) [59,60,61]. Some of them showed better efficacy against pyrazinamide-resistant strains, but there is no data or references about anti MDR-TB activity.

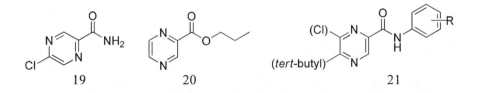

19   20   21

Galactose and arabinose are predominant in the cell wall mainly as arabino-D-galactan and lipoarabinomannans. Glycosyl transferases are intricately involved in the biosynthesis of these polymers. *Ethambutol*, an amino alcohol well known as an anti-TB drug presently used in clinics as a first-line agent, acts through inhibition of arabinosyl transferases. The galactopyranosyl amino alcohols were synthesised and screened for antitubercular activities. The compounds, where two galactopyranosyl units are linked by a longer carbon chain, showed potent activity against *Mycobacterium tuberculosis* $H_{37}Rv$. The compound with 1-[12-(2-hydroxypropylamino)dodecylamino]propan-2-ol moiety (22; n – 12) demonstrated *in vitro* MIC of 1.56 µg/mL and also displayed activity in MDR-TB. The compound was found to be superior to ethambutol in *in vitro* screening [62,63].

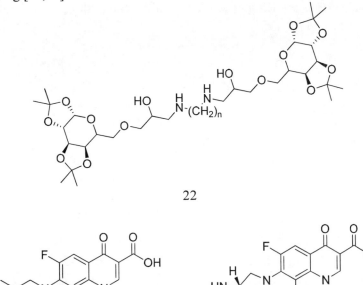

22

23   24

Fluoroquinolones of the fourth generation, such as gatifloxacin (23) and moxifloxacin (24), act by the inhibiting DNA topoisomerase IV and DNA gyrase. They have a longer half-life and exhibit the highest *in vitro* activity against *M. tbc.* with MIC_{90} 0.031-0.125 µg/mL [64,65]. They were found to kill rifampicin-tolerant bacteria more effectively than levofloxacin or ofloxacin, may possess the sterilising activity [66], and have the potential to shorten the TB therapy which represents a major advance [67]. They could have the potential to be used as first-line drugs to improve treatment of TB. Moxifloxacin might be very useful against MDR-TB since it has no cross-resistance to other anti-tuberculosis drug classes. When tested against 86 strains of *M. tbc.*, including 13 resistant and 4 multidrug-resistant ones, moxifloxacin was effective against all strains at 0.5 µg/mL, except two multidrug-resistant strains, which have MIC = 2 and > 4 µg/mL, respectively [68].

Sitafloxacin (25) hydrate (DU-6859a, Gracevit), a new-generation, broad-spectrum oral fluoroquinolone is very active against many Gram-positive, Gram-negative, and anaerobic clinical isolates, including strains resistant to other fluoroquinolones [69]. Minimum inhibitory concentrations of gemifloxacin (26) were determined for 40 available multidrug-resistant *M. tbc.* isolates in Taiwan [70].

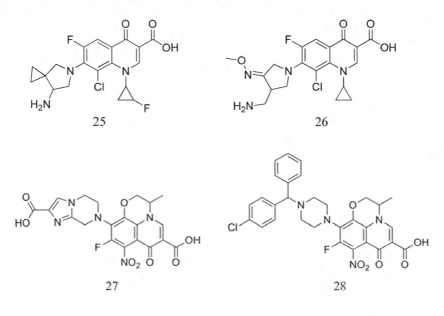

Novel ofloxacin derivatives were synthesised and evaluated for *in vitro* and *in vivo* activities against *Mycobacterium tuberculosis* H$_{37}$Rv, multidrug-resistant *M. tbc.*, *M. smegmatis* and tested for the ability to inhibit the supercoiling activity of DNA gyrase from mycobacteria. 10-[2-Carboxy-5,6-dihydroimidazo[1,2-*a*]pyrazin-7(8*H*)-yl]-9-fluoro-2,3-dihydro-3-methyl-8-nitro-7-oxo-3,7-dihydro-2*H*-[1,4]oxazino[2,3,4-*ij*]quinoline-6-carboxylic acid (27) was found to be the most active compound *in vitro* with MIC$_{99}$ of 0.19 µM and 0.09 µM against *M. tbc.* and MDR-TB, respectively. In the *in vivo* animal model, the same compound also decreased the bacterial load in the lung and spleen tissues with 1.91 and 2.91 log protections, respectively, at the dose of 50 mg/kg body weight. Compound 10-{4-[(4-chlorophenyl)(phenyl)-

methyl]piperazin-1-yl}-9-fluoro-3-methyl-8-nitro-7-oxo-3,7-dihydro-2*H*-[1,4]-oxazino[2,3,4-*ij*]quinoline-6-carboxylic acid (28) was detected to be the most active in the inhibition of the supercoiling activity of DNA gyrase with IC_{50} of 10.0 µg/mL. The results demonstrate the potential and importance of developing new oxazino quinolone derivatives against mycobacterial infections [71].

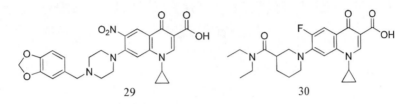

29   30

A group of newly prepared 1-(substituted)-1,4-dihydro-6-nitro-4-oxo-7-(substituent; secondary amino)-quinoline-3-carboxylic acids was evaluated in the same way. 7-{4-[(Benzo[*d*][1,3]dioxol-5-yl)methyl]piperazin-1-yl}-1-cyclopropyl-6-nitro-4-oxo-1,4-dihydroquinoline-3-carboxylic acid (29) was found as the most active compound *in vitro* with MIC of 0.08 and 0.16 µM against *M. tbc.*, MDR-TB (resistant to isoniazid, rifampicin, ethambutol and ofloxacin) and *M. smegmatis*. With respect to the structure-activity relationship, results demonstrated that N^1-cyclopropyl is favourable for anti-mycobacterial activity, analogously to clinically-used quinolones. For the substitution on C-7 was optimal substituted piperazine. The named compound was tested *in vivo* in the dose of 50 mg/kg and it decreased the bacterial load in lung and spleen tissues with 2.78 and 4.15 log protections, respectively, and was considered to be promising in reducing the bacterial count in lung and spleen tissues. The inhibition of the supercoiling activity of *M. smegmatis* DNA gyrase showed that 7-{4-[(benzo[*d*][1,3]dioxol-5-yl)methyl]piperazin-1-yl}-1-cyclopropyl-6-nitro-4-oxo-1,4-dihydroquinoline-3-carboxylic   acid inhibits this enzyme at a concentration of 30 µg/mL [72]. 6-Nitro group could be replaced by 6-fluoro group without loss of anti-mycobacterial activity. Tested strains were the same as we mentioned above. Among the synthesized compounds, 1-cyclopropyl-7-[3-(diethylcarbamoyl)piperidin-1-yl]-6-fluoro-4-oxo-1,4-dihydroquinoline-3 carboxylic acid (30) was described as the most active *in vitro* with MIC of 0.09 µM against *M. tbc.* and MDR-TB. *In vivo* in the animal model, it decreased the mycobacterial load in lung and spleen tissues with 2.53 and 4.88 log protections, respectively, at a dose of 50 mg/kg body weight. This compound has an IC_{50} value of supercoiling activity of DNA gyrase of 100 µg/mL [73].

2. NEW LEADS WITH NOVEL MECHANISM OF THE ACTION [74] (LINEZOLID, TMC207, PA-824, OPC-67683, BM212, SQ109, FAS20013, LL-3858)

Oxazolidinones represented by (*S*)-*N*-{[3-(3-fluoro-4-morpholinophenyl)-2-oxooxazolidin-5-yl]methyl}acetamide (*linezolid*; 31) [75,76,77,78] are a new class of antibiotics. Linezolid is used for the treatment of infections caused by multi-resistant bacteria including streptococci and methicillin-resistant *Staphylococcus aureus* (MRSA). It is marketed by Pfizer under the trade name Zyvox (in the United States and several other countries), Zyvoxam (in Canada and Mexico), or Zyvoxid (in Europe). Linezolid has been also used to treat tuberculosis [79]. The optimal dose for the use in tuberculosis is not known. In adults, 600 mg daily [80] or 600 mg twice daily [81] have both been used with good effect. The mechanism of the action for inhibiting microbial protein synthesis is unique: targeting microbial protein synthesis – either the 30S or the 70S ribosomal initiation complex [82,83]. Its thiomorpholine analogue, *PNU-100480* (32), was also active against drug-resistant strains of *M. tbc.* (MIC ≤ 0.5-4 µg/mL). It is well absorbed and tolerated in animal models [84].

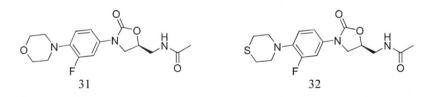

31   32

The tetrazole-bearing oxazolidinones such as *DA-7867* (Dong-A Pharmaceutical Co., Yongin, Korea; 33) are new hetero-ring-substituted pyridine-containing oxazolidinones, (*S*)-*N*-[(3-{3-fluoro-4-[6-(1-methyl-1*H*-tetrazol-5-yl)pyridin-3-yl]phenyl}-2-oxooxazolidin-5-yl)methyl]acetamide. It is more active *in vitro* against *M. tuberculosis* isolates than linezolid, with a MIC range from 0.03 to 0.5 µg/mL [85]. Even if linezolid and DA-7867 are structurally quite similar, they have different pharmacokinetics in mice. After 4 hours, the levels of linezolid are very low, and that can explain the low level of activity in the mouse model. On the other hand, mouse plasma levels of DA-7867 remain higher than those of linezolid and R207910, which makes this drug a good candidate to be tested in animal models.

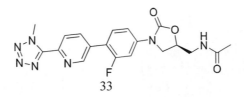

33

Diarylquinoline drug candidate *TMC207*, or J (previously R207910; 34), owned by Johnson & Johnson, has many characteristics that make it an attractive TB drug candidate, including low molecular weight, high potency against drug-sensitive and drug-resistant TB strains, very long half-life (permitting once-weekly dosing), and low potential for drug interactions. It exhibits an excellent activity against both drug-sensitive and drug-resistant *M. tbc.* with MIC 0.06 µg/mL [86]. It has also a great potency against mutated drug-resistant strains, MDR and XDR *M. tbc.* strain, with no cross-resistance to the current first-line drugs [87]. The use of TMC207 alone appears to be at least as effective as a combination of RIF, INH, and PZA and more effective than RIF alone in mouse models. [74] The unique mechanism of the action, inhibition of mycobacterial membrane-bound ATP-synthase offers great potential because there is little similarity between the mycobacterial and human proteins encoded by the *atpE* gene that code for the c subunit of ATP-synthase, which has been identified as the specific target of TMC207 [88]. Synergic activity was observed with PZA [89], and, when associated with PZA, RIF, and moxifloxacin, it shortened the duration of the treatment [90]. Mutations of *atpE* are responsible for resistance to diarylquinoline [52]. The unique dual bactericidal activity of diarylquinolines on dormant as well as replicating bacterial subpopulations distinguishes them entirely from the current anti-tuberculosis drugs and underlines the potential of TMC207 to shorten tuberculosis treatment [91]. Therefore, it is the most promising drug candidate in the last 30 years.

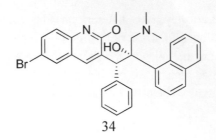

34

The lead compound from a group of bicyclic nitroimidazopyrans, nitroimidazo[2,1-*b*]oxazine *PA-824* (undergoing Phase II clinical trials; 35), is active against replicating (aerobic) and non-replicating (anaerobic) mycobacteria [92]. PA-824 causes an accumulation of hydroxymycolic acids by the inhibition of an enzyme that oxidizes hydroxymycolate to ketomycolate. In fact, it is a prodrug metabolized before it can exert its effect. Its MIC against *M. tbc.* is 0.015-0.25 µg/mL and PA-824 is equally active against mono- and multi-resistant strains without cross-resistance with current anti-tubercular drugs [93]. It may be used in combination with RIF to accelerate the killing of persisting *M. tbc.*, moreover, to shorten the duration of TB therapy [94]. PA-824 in combination with isoniazid prevents the selection of TB mutants resistant to isoniazid [95]. Unlike current TB drugs, it has shown high bactericidal activity against all MDR-TB isolates as well as potential for activity against latent strains.

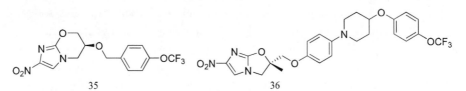

35   36

Another derivative, (*S*)-2-methyl-6-nitro-2-{4-[4-(4-trifluoromethoxy)-piperidin-1-yl]phenoxymethyl}-2,3-dihydroimidazo[2,1-*b*]oxazole *OPC-67683* (36), is also in Phase II clinical trials. It has from 6- to 7-fold stronger activity than the first-line anti-tuberculous drugs RIF or INH with MIC 0.006-0.024 µg/mL against *M. tbc.* The compound exhibits excellent *in vitro* activity against drug-susceptible and resistant *M. tbc.* strains and does not show cross-resistance to any current first-line drugs [96]. The long half-life of OPC-67683, the lack of metabolization by CYP enzymes and its efficacy in immunocompromised mice suggest that this drug may be useful for the treatment of co-infected TB/HIV patients [74]. The cell wall is the target of the action. It inhibits like INH methoxymycolic and ketomycolic acid synthesis at significantly lower concentrations, but does not inhibit α-mycolic acid biosynthesis. As in the case of PA-824, OPC-67683 is also a prodrug. *Mycobacterium tuberculosis* metabolises the drug and produces one main metabolite, a desnitroimidazooxazole. Both these compounds show potential as anti-persistence drugs, although their hydrophobic nature may lead to bioavailability problems in humans, so the results of ADME and toxicity tests are important [97].

The class under Italian investigation is based on 1,5-diaryl-2-methyl-3-(4-methylpiperazin-1-yl)methylpyrrol ring. Among these compounds, the pyrrol derivative *BM212* (37) appeared the most potent against both drug-resistant and intramacrophagic mycobacteria with MIC between 0.7 and 1.5 μg/mL [98]. A series of BM212 derivatives was made in order to improve potency. Among these, a thiomorpholine derivative (38) was found to be more potent and less toxic than BM212, with MIC 0.4 μg/mL [99,100,101].

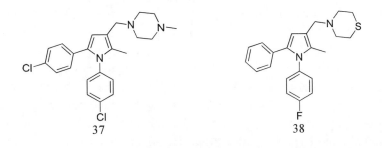

37   38

The synthesis and screening of diamine analogues of ethambutol has yielded a library of compounds having an ethylenediamine pharmacophore. The generated *N*-geranyl-*N*′-(2-adamantyl)ethane-1,2-diamine (SQ109; 39) displayed an excellent *in vitro* activity against *M. tbc.* (MIC 0.16-0.64 μg/mL) [102,103], including the strains resistant to EMB, INH, and RIF. SQ109 appears to be rapidly metabolized in the liver and is probably a prodrug [104]. The exact mechanism is not known, although it is believed to target cell wall synthesis in a different manner than EMB because SQ109 is active against EMB-resistant strains [105]. The combined administration of SQ109 and RIF, INH, or PZA exhibits synergic *in vitro* activity and is also potent against RIF-resistant strains [106]. SQ109 displays a 14- to 35-fold improvement in activity compared to EMB.

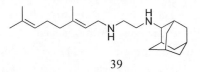

39

Sulfonyl acetamides as transition-state analogues of beta-ketoacyl synthase reaction showed 2-(decylsulfonyl)acetamide (FAS20013; 40) being the most active. FAS20013 exhibits MIC 0.71-1.5 µg/mL, though it may also interfere with ATP synthesis of *M. tbc*. FAS20013 is characterized as an ideal anti-TB agent based on compelling new findings. Its potent killing activity is directed specifically against slow growing mycobacteria that cause the disease rather than at a broad array of non-pathogenic organisms, which merely enhance the emergence of drug-resistant strains. No resistance has been encountered to FAS20013 in clinical isolates, nor have resistant organisms been induced in the laboratory despite multiple attempts. The short-term killing power of FAS20013 is greater than currently used drugs; for example, FAS20013 will kill more organisms in a 4-hour exposure than isoniazid or rifampicin can during a 12- to 14-day exposure. The compound is very effective in killing MDR-TB organisms that are resistant to multiple drugs now in use. A series of recent laboratory experiments indicates the superior effect to current drugs of FAS20013´s ability to "sterilize" TB lesions and kill the TB organisms surviving in the latent infections that exist in one-third of the world´s population. Therapeutic evaluation of FAS20013 in a model TB infection in mice has repeatedly shown its effectiveness as well as freedom from adverse side effects. The compound is up to 100% orally bio-available. To date, no dose-limiting toxicity has been encountered, even when doses 10 times the effective dose were administered.

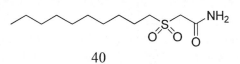

40

FAS20013 inhibits biosynthesis of the mycolic acids and appears to interfere with a vital step in the organism's energy generating metabolic pathways. This mechanism differs from all drugs currently used to treat tuberculosis.

Pyrrol *LL-3858* (41) (additional name Sudoterb) was approved for preclinical testing in Lupin Ltd. [107,108]. The compound belongs to a class of plant alkaloids with INH moiety. LL-3858 has activity *in vitro* and *in vivo*. *In vitro* it has bactericidal activity similar to INH (MIC 0.025-0.12 μg/mL) and is synergic with RIF. A combination with INH, RIF, and PZA led to the complete sterilization of both sensitive and MDR strains in mice within two months in combination with RIF- and PZA-cured TB in all animals after 3 months. The compound exhibits good oral bio-availability with once daily dosing.

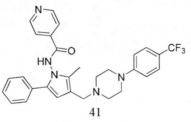

41

3. NOVEL DRUG TARGETS [109]

A variety of different approaches exist to the discovery of new anti-infective agents. During the last several years, more emphasis has been placed on the target-based methods in which an essential protein, usually an enzyme, is used in high-throughput screens of libraries.

Current TB drugs inhibit particular targets in DNA synthesis, RNA synthesis, cell wall synthesis, and energy metabolism pathways (Table 2). Mycobacterial two-component systems, sigma factors, and virulence factors have also been proposed as targets for TB drug development. Novel targets such as essential genes, persistence targets, toxin-antitoxin modules, and energy-production pathways are the choice of targets [52].

3.1. Cell Wall Biosynthesis

The mycobacterial cell wall is a lipid barrier formed from three main components—peptidoglycan, arabinogalactan and mycolic acids—that are not found in mammalian cells. Their biosynthesis offers an attractive target for the development of new drugs.

One of the key enzymes, InhA, the enoyl acyl-carrier protein reductase is involved in the mycobacterial fatty acid elongation cycle. InhA is a superb target for future drug development since compounds that do not require activation should be able to be developed. There are approximately 250 identified genes [110] related to the biosynthesis of the lipid turnover that contain InhA, the main target of INH. Thus, the logical approach for developing a chemotherapy agent against tubercle bacilli includes screening compounds that could inhibit the biosynthesis of mycolic acids.

Cell Wall Structure of M. Tuberculosis [111]

The structure of the *M. tuberculosis* cell wall is very specific and special. The mycobacterial cell wall is extraordinarily thick and tight, having three main components:

1) characteristic long-chain fatty acids, mycolic acids,
2) unique polysaccharides, arabinogalactans (AG) that are esterified by mycolic acids,
3) peptidoglycan (PG), which is attached to AG via a phosphodiester bridge.

The mycolyl-AG complex is attached to the peptidoglycan, a porous layer between the wall and the plasma membrane, and form the mycolyl-AG peptidoglycan complex. The mycobacterial cell wall also contains many "free" lipid species, called extractable lipids that are not covalently linked to the AG-peptidoglycan complex and are solvent-extractable. The free lipids include glycolipids, phenolic glycolipids, glycopeptolipids, and other chemical species [112] (Figure 4).

Mycobacterial mycolic acids (Figure 5) have several distinctive features compared to most fatty acids: they are long-chain β-hydroxy acids having an α-carbon-long branch. The main chain of 40-60 carbons has very few double bonds or cyclopropyl groups and the short α-branch is totally saturated typically of 24 carbons. The long chain has only two positions that are observed to be occupied by functional groups. Of these two positions, the proximal position (nearer the β-hydroxy moiety) contains exclusively *cis-* or *trans*-olefin or a cyclopropane ring, while the distal position may be the same as the proximal position or may contain one of a variety of oxygen moieties such as α-methyl ketone, α-methyl ether, methyl-branched ester, or α-methyloxirane.

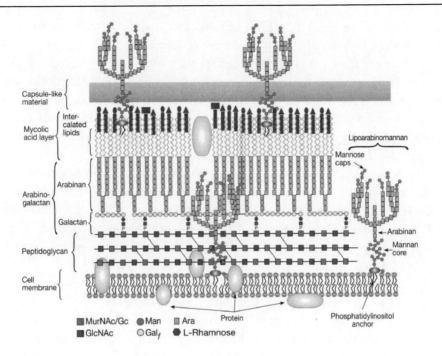

Figure 4. Structure of mycolyl-AG-peptidoglycan complex (this picture was taken from [113]).

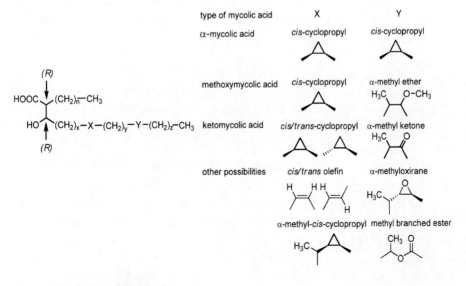

Figure 5. Mycolic acid general structure

The usual value for n is 23. The sum of x, y, and z is approximately 50. Both α and β carbons of mycolic acid have R chirality.

There are three kinds of mycolates, α-mycolates, methoxymycolates, and ketomycolates. Both the α- and methoxymycolates only have the *cis*-cyclopropyl group at the proximal position, while 17% of cyclopropyl groups at the keto proximal position are *trans*. 51% of the total mycolates are α-mycolates, 36% are methoxymycolates, and 13% are ketomycolates. All three mycolates contain 24 and 26 carbon α branches in approximately the *ratio* of 10:90, with negligible amounts of 22 carbons α-branches. Methoxymycolates and ketomycolates have longer main chains than α-mycolates. The total carbon numbers for the α-, methoxy and keto forms are 76-82, 83-90, and 84-89, respectively. The differences in mycolic acid structure may affect the fluidity and permeability of bilayer, and may explain the different sensitivity levels of various mycobacterial species to lipophilic inhibitors.

AG, the other main component of a mycobacterial cell wall, is a polysaccharide consisting of arabinose and galactose. Within AG, all arabinose and galactose residues are in the furanose form, and mycolic acids are located in clusters of four on the terminal hexaarabinofuranoside through 1.5 linkages. However, only two-thirds of terminal arabinose residues are mycolated. The linker disaccharide phosphate connects the galactan region of AG to peptidoglycan [112]. The enzymes that are involved in the biosynthesis of the mycobacterial cell wall offer attractive targets for the development of new drugs.

3.1.1. Mycolic Acid Synthesis Inhibitors

Phenazinamine derivatives closely related to the anti-leprosy drug clofazimine, (*E*)-*N*,5-bis(4-chlorophenyl)-3-(isopropylimino)-3,5-dihydro-phenazin-2-amine (CFM; 42), are active against a range of clinical *M. tbc.* isolates including MDR strains [114].

Clofazimine and its derivatives stimulate intracellular hydrogen peroxide production and inhibit the multiplication of cells because of binding to the guanine in DNA [115]. More recently, it was described that dihydrophenazine derivatives showed dose-dependent inhibitory activity against mycolic acid biosynthesis [116].

Reddy et al. [117] referred that the anti-tuberculous activity of clofazimine and its two derivatives B4154 (43) and B4157 (44) were selected as a more convenient form of other clofazimine analogues. These three compounds have been assessed on twenty *M. tuberculosis* strains, including 7 single drug-resistant strains (resistant to RIF, INH, or EMB) and 7 MDR strains. All of these strains were susceptible to B4154 and B4157, and only one MDR strain showed moderate resistance to clofazimine. MIC_{90} of B4154, B4157, and CFM were 0.25, 0.12, and ≤ 1.0 μg/mL, respectively, and the intracellular activities in macrophages of CFM and B4157 were superior to B4154. The anti-mycobacterial activities were evaluated *in vivo* in C57BL/6 mice, too. At a dose of 20 mg/kg of body weight, the activity of CFM was slightly superior to B4157, but both compounds prevented mortality and caused a significant reduction in the numbers of CFU in the lungs and spleens comparable to isoniazid or rifampicin. This clofazimine derivatives show additional pharmacological activities – pro-oxidative by stimulation of superoxide anion production and stimulation of phospholipase A_2, and some compounds including CFM reversed the inhibitory effect of the mycobacterial proteins on phagocytic function and showed anti-inflammatory properties [115].

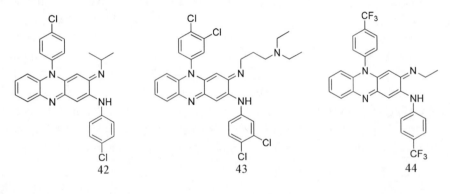

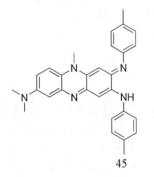

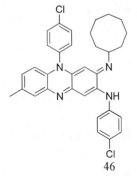

Compound (45), a new dihydrophenazine derivative (E)-N^8,N^8,5-trimethyl-N^2-p-tolyl-3-(p-tolylimino)-3,5-dihydrophenazine-2,8-diamine, possesses a unique profile. Many derivatives of this compound were synthesized and one candidate, *OPC-37306* (46) ((E)-N,5-bis(4-chlorophenyl)-3-(cyclooctylimino)-8-methyl-3,5-dihydrophenazin-2-amine), showed dose-dependent inhibitory activity against mycolic biosynthesis with MIC in the range from 0.1 to 0.2 µg/mL against *M. tbc.*-resistant strains to INH, RIF, EMB, STM, *M. tbc.* Kurono, and *M. bovis* BCG. The interesting fact was that compound did not kill Gram-positive bacteria or Gram-negative bacteria [116].

Fatty acid biosynthesis [118]
One of the fatty acid synthase inhibitors is cerulenin (47), a natural product from *Cephalosporium caerulens*. It inhibits both type I and II fatty acid synthases. It has been previously shown that cerulenin, in addition, has synergistic effects when used with rifampicin, isoniazid, ofloxacin, amikacin, and clofazimine *in vitro*. More recently, cerulenin has been shown to be inhibitory to a range of mycobacteria including resistant *M. tuberculosis* (resistant to one or more of the following drugs – isoniazid, rifampicin, ethambutol, streptomycin, and pyrazinamide, including one strain resistant to all five of the first-line anti-tuberculotics) with MIC ranging from 1.5 to 12.5 µg/mL and several non-tuberculous mycobacteria. Cerulenin itself is an unstable compound in mammalian organisms, but the inhibition of fatty acid synthesis is a potential new target for anti-mycobacterial therapy [119,120].

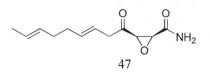

47

DesA3
DesA3 is a membrane-bound stearoyl-CoA Δ^9-desaturase that produces oleic acid, a precursor of mycobacterial membrane phospholipids and triglycerides. DesA3 has sequence homology with other membrane desaturases including the presence of the eight His motifs proposed to bind the diiron centre active site. This family of desaturases functions as multi-component complexes, and thus requires electron transfer proteins for efficient catalytic turnover. Rv3230c from *Mycobacterium tuberculosis* $H_{37}Rv$ is a

biologically-relevant electron transfer partner for DesA3 from the same pathogen. Rv3230c was expressed as a partially-soluble protein in *Escherichia coli*; recombinant DesA3 was expressed in *Mycobacterium smegmatis* as a catalytically-active membrane protein. The addition of *E. coli* lysates containing Rv3230c to lysates of *M. smegmatis* expressing DesA3 gave strong conversion of [1-^{14}C]-18.0-CoA to [1-^{14}C]-*cis*-Δ^9-18:1-CoA and of [1-^{14}C]-16:0-CoA to [1-^{14}C]-*cis*-Δ^9-16:1-CoA. Both *M. tuberculosis* proteins were required to reconstitute activity, as various combinations of control lysates lacking either Rv3230c or DesA3 gave minimal or no activity [121,122].

The thiourea isoxyl (thiocarlide, ISO; 1,3-bis[4-(isopentyloxy)-phenyl]thiourea) is known to be an effective anti-tuberculosis drug active against a range of multidrug-resistant strains of *Mycobacterium tuberculosis* and has been used clinically. Isoxyl inhibits a stearoylcoenzyme A desaturase (DesA3), an enzyme responsible for the insertion of a double bond at carbon-9 of stearic acid [123,124]. ISO is a prodrug requiring prior metabolic activation for anti-mycobacterial activity. The same role of EthA (a flavin monooxygenase) is for oxidation of ethionamide to the sulfinic acid, which is further transformed to amide (Figure 6) [125].

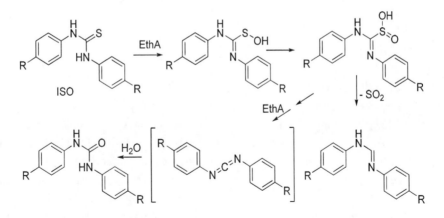

Figure 6. Metabolic conversion of isoxyl.

A series of its derivatives and other urea derivatives (48, 49, 50, 51) was synthesised to improve the activity [126].

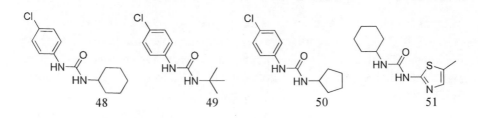

          48   49   50   51

Related to these compounds are thiourea derivatives. Based on structural similarity, it is possible that this group is acting by the same mechanisms as isoxyl. New 1-(5-cyclobutyl-1,3-oxazol-2-yl)-3-(substituted)phenyl/pyridyl thioureas were evaluated *in vitro* and *in vivo* against *M. tbc.* H₃₇Rv and a clinical isolate of MDR-TB. Seven compounds inhibited both *M. tbc.* and MDR-TB *in vitro* with MIC of < 1 μM. The most active was found 1-(5-cyclobutyloxazol-2-yl)-3-[(2-(trifluoromethyl)phenyl]thiourea (52) with an *in vitro* MIC of 0.14 μM and was 2.5 and 80 times more active than isoniazid against *M. tbc.* and MDR-TB, respectively. The compound was non-toxic to Vero cells up to 183 μM, with a selectivity index of > 1307 [127].

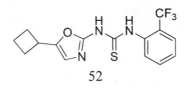

                                    52

3.1.2. Protein Synthesis Inhibitors [119]

Peptide deformylase (PDF) catalyzes the hydrolytic removal of the *N*-terminal formyl group from nascent proteins. This is an essential step in bacterial protein synthesis, making PDF an attractive target for antibacterial drug development. Essentiality of the *def* gene, encoding PDF from *Mycobacterium tuberculosis* was demonstrated through genetic knockout experiments with *Mycobacterium bovis* BCG. PDF from *M. tbc.* strain H₃₇Rv was cloned, expressed, and purified as an *N*-terminal histidine-tagged recombinant protein in *Escherichia coli*. A novel class of PDF inhibitors (PDF-I), derived of *N*-alkyl urea hydroxamic acids [128], was synthesized and evaluated for their activities against the *M. tbc.* PDF enzyme, as well as their anti-mycobacterial effects. Several compounds from the new class had 50% inhibitory concentration (IC₅₀) values of < 100 μM. Some of the PDF-I displayed antibacterial activity against *M. tbc.*, including MDR strains with MIC₉₀ values of < 1 μM. Pharmacokinetic studies of potential leads showed that the compounds were orally bio-available. Spontaneous resistance towards these inhibitors arose at a frequency of $\leq 5 \times 10^{-7}$ in *M. bovis* BCG. DNA sequence analysis of several spontaneous PDF-I-resistant mutants revealed that half of the mutants had acquired point mutations in their formyl methyltransferase gene (*fmt*), which formylated Met-tRNA. The results validate *M. tuberculosis* PDF as a drug target and suggest that this class of compounds has the potential to be developed as novel anti-mycobacterial agents [129]. The analogues of the most active *LBK-611* (PGΓ 611; 53), (*S*)-1-{(*R*)-2-[(*N*-hydroxyformamido)methyl]hexanoyl}-*N*-(pyridin-2-yl)pyrrolidine-2-carboxamide, having benzimidazole or benzoxazole moiety (54; MBG means metal-binding group, R = alkyl, Y = O, NH) were prepared and evaluated. The nature of the chelating group has been found to be very important for the effect on *M. tbc.* PDF activity. Carboxylic acids are significantly less active than corresponding hydroxamic acids and reverse hydroxamic acids (same for LBK-611). The activity depends on the chelating properties [130].

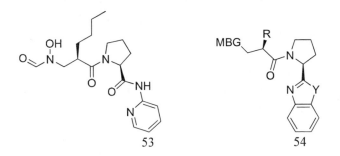

53   54

Inhibition of InhA

InhA, an enoyl acyl-carrier protein reductase, is the key enzyme involved in the type II fatty acid elongation cycle (Figure 2). Inhibition of InhA disrupts the biosynthesis of the mycolic acids that are central constituents of the mycobacterial cell. However, the biochemical and functional differences between the bacterial and mammal's fatty acid synthetic pathway are due to the mycobacterial enzymes with distinct properties. Therefore, inhibitors targeting InhA directly without a requirement for activation would be promising candidates for the development of agents against the ever-increasing threat from drug-resistant *Mycobacterium tuberculosis* strains. It has been validated as an effective antimicrobial target. Discovery and optimization of pyrrolidine carboxamides as a novel series of direct InhA inhibitors reveals effective candidates. Compounds with a single electron-withdrawing substituent at the *meta*-position of an aromatic ring (*i.e.* (*R*)-1-cyclohexyl-*N*-(3,5-dichlorophenyl)-5-oxopyrrolidine-3-carboxamide) are the most potent inhibitors (Figure 7) [131].

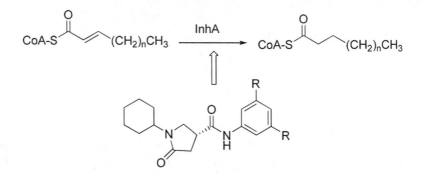

Figure 7. Mechanisms of the action of (*R*)-1-cyclohexyl-*N*-(3,5-dichlorophenyl)-5-oxopyrrolidine-3-carboxamides.

Direct InhA inhibitors do not require mycobacterial enzymatic activation, thus circumventing the resistance mechanism that is observed in drug-resistant clinical isolates. A novel class of InhA inhibitors based on an arylamide series of compounds containing piperazine or piperidine (55) as the core structure was evaluated; the best activity has shown [4-(3-chlorophenyl)piperazin-1-yl](2,4-dimethylphenyl)methanone (56) [132].

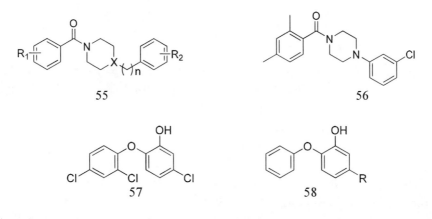

McMurry and co-workers [133] were the first who provided evidence that triclosan (57) targets the FabI enoyl reductase enzyme in the bacterial FAS II pathway. Triclosan has a MIC_{99} value of 12.5 µg/mL (43 µM) for $H_{37}Rv$, which decreases to 3.8 and 1 µg/mL (17.5 and 3.5 µM) for the diphenyl ethers (58) with 5-ethyl (2PP) and 5-pentyl (5PP) substituents, respectively. However, when the alkyl chain was extended to 14 carbons, a much larger MIC_{99} value of 175 µg/mL (460 µM) was obtained. Triclosan, 6PP and 8PP were also evaluated against five clinical tuberculous strains and were each shown to have MIC_{99} values close to those exhibited against $H_{37}Rv$. In contrast, while the MIC_{99} values for INH against three of the clinical strains (W210, NHN20, and HN335) were similar to the value obtained against $H_{37}Rv$ (0.05 µg/mL, 0.37 µM), strains TN587 and NHN382 had MIC_{99} values 30-50-fold higher than for $H_{37}Rv$. Thus, not only are 6PP and 8PP more potent than triclosan at inhibiting the growth of *M. tuberculosis*, but they are also active against clinical strains resistant to the front line TB drug INH. In support of the hypothesis, InhA inhibitors that do not require KatG activation are active against the INH-resistant mycobacterial strain [134]. Diphenyl ether-based InhA inhibitors do not require activation by the mycobacterial KatG enzyme, thereby circumventing the normal mechanism of resistance to the front line drug isoniazid (INH), and thus accounting for their activity against INH-resistant tuberculous strains.

Heterocyclic ortho-fused diazaborines (59) were found to be inhibitors of InhA, the enoyl-ACP reductase [135]. They inhibit FabI via the formation of a covalent bond between the boron atom and the 2′-hydroxyl of the NAD^+ ribose. The diazaborine group binds in the active site where the enoyl substrate is normally located, and thus the diazaborine-NAD adduct is a bisubstrate FabI inhibitor. SAR studies have shown that the diaza-moiety and the boron atom are essential for the activity [136].

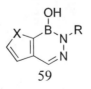

59

3.1.3. Polysaccharide Biosynthesis Inhibitors [137]

Arabinofuranosides constitute one of the important components of cell wall structures of mycobacteria. With this importance of arabinofuranosides in mind, alkyl glycosides bearing arabinofuranoside trisaccharides were prepared, wherein the sugars were presented either in the monovalent or bivalent forms. Following the synthesis, the monovalent and bivalent alkyl glycosides were tested for their activities in a mycobacterial growth assay. The growth of the mycobacterial strain *M. smegmatis* was assessed in the presence of the alkyl glycosides and it was realized that the alkyl glycosides acted as inhibitors of the mycobacterial growth. The inhibition of the growth, caused by the above alkyl glycosides, was not observed for the arabinofuranose trisaccharide alone, without the alkyl groups, and for an alkyl glycoside-bearing maltose as the sugar component [138].

A series of α-(1→6)-linked mannose disaccharides in which the 2'-OH group has been replaced, independently, by deoxy, fluoro, amino, and methoxy functionalities (60; R = H, F, NH$_2$, OCH$_3$) has been synthesized. Evaluation of these compounds as potential substrates or inhibitors of a polyprenol monophosphomannose-dependent α-(1→6)-mannosyltransferase involved in mycobacterial lipoarabinomannan (LAM) biosynthesis demonstrated that the enzyme is a somewhat tolerant substitution at this site. LAM is the major antigenic component of the cell wall and has been implicated in a large and increasing number of important immunological events. The enzyme recognizes the disaccharides with groups similar or smaller than the native hydroxyl, but not the disaccharide with the more sterically-demanding methoxy group. The 2'-OH appears not to form a critical hydrogen bonding interaction with the protein as the 2'-deoxy analogue is a substrate for the enzyme [139].

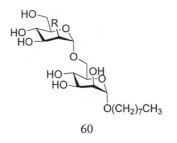

60

The *Mycobacterium tuberculosis* MEP (2C-methyl-D-erythritol 4-phosphate) pathway promises bacterium-specific drug targets for new drugs [140]. All isoprenoids are derived from the repetitive condensation of two important precursors, isopentenyl diphosphate (IPP) and dimethylallyl diphosphate (DMAPP), catalyzed by prenyl diphosphate synthetases. In *M. tbc.*, IPP and DMAPP are biosynthesized only through the 2C-methyl-Derythrol 4-phosphate pathway [141]. A number of isoprenoids have been observed and characterized in *M. tbc.* including polyprenyl phosphate (Pol-P), the prenyl side-chain of menaquinone and various forms of carotenoids. Pol-P is involved in the biosynthesis of arabinogalactan, arabinomannan, lipoarabinomannan, and other lipids of peptidoglycan biosynthesis. It plays a critical role in cell wall biosynthesis as a lipid carrier of the active sugars. Therefore, the MEP pathway can be considered as a potential source of novel drug targets [142].

Since peptidoglycan is an essential bacterial cell wall polymer, peptidoglycan biosynthesis provides a unique and selective target for the mechanism of the action of bacteria. Phospho-*N*-acetylmuramyl-pentapeptide translocase (translocase I) is an integral membrane protein that catalyzes the first step of the intramembrane cycle of reactions involved in peptidoglycan assembly. In the course of screening for new antibiotics with translocase I inhibitory activity, there was identified a series of capuramycin analogues that proved to have selective antibacterial activity against mycobacteria. Capuramycin analogue *RS-118641* (61) was the most potent compound overall. The MIC$_{50/90}$ (µg/mL) results for RS-118641 were: *M. tbc.* 1/2; MDR *M. tbc.* 0.5/2; *M. avium* 4/8; and *M. intracellulare* 0.06/0.5 [143]. These results suggest that capuramycin analogues exhibit strong anti-mycobacterial potential and are excellent candidates for further evaluation in the treatment of *M. tuberculosis* and MDR infections in humans.

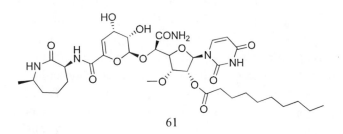

61

Nitrofuranylamides
N-(3-chloro-4-methoxyphenyl)-5-nitrofuran-2-carboxamide (first lead) was selected as the anti-tuberculosis agent with a novel mechanism of the action active on both growing and latent bacteria. Cell wall biosynthetic cascade is an ideal target selection criterion. Arabinogalactan, an essential component of the tuberculosis cell wall, contains galactofuranose building blocks, which are not found in the human host. UDP-galactose mutase (Glf) is

a flavin dependant enzyme, which catalyzes the conversion of UDP-galactofuranose from UDP-galactopyranose.

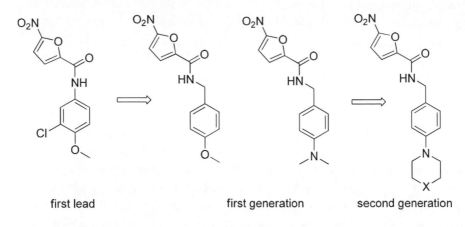

first lead   first generation   second generation

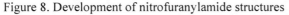

Figure 8. Development of nitrofuranylamide structures

The nitrofuranylamide was identified as an inhibitor of Glf. Its MIC = 1.6 µg/mL [144]. Optimization and development of convenient form having good activity, solubility, and bio-availability led to the library of the first and the second generation (Figure 8; X = O, NH, N-Me, N-benzyl, CH-benzyl, S, SO, SO_2, N-pyridin-2-yl).

Amides derived from benzylamines have greater MIC_{90} activity than the amides derived from anilines. The methoxy substitution on the *para*-position of the benzyl group was very favourable compared to the *ortho* and *meta* positions. The extension of a functional group replacement strategy at the *para* position led to the introduction of the dimethylamino group. The methylamine analogue retained the same MIC_{90} activity of 0.1 µg/mL as a methoxy derivative and increased solubility by the salt formulation. The nitro group and furan ring have been determined essential for activity. The inspiration for the second-generation development has brought about the development of the fluoroquinolones. During the development of norfloxacin from the first generation quinolones, the bio-availability of the series was significantly boosted by the introduction of piperazine moiety at the 7-position of the quinolone core. Based on this strategy, substituted cyclic secondary amine instead of *N,N*-dimethyl group was introduced. In a second generation, the most active cyclic secondary amine *N*-[4-(4-*N*-benzylpiperazin-1-yl)benzyl]-5-nitrofuran-2-carboxamide (62) has shown activity in MIC_{90} 0.0125 µg/mL and its fluoro derivative (63) showed MIC$_{90}$ of 0.025 µg/mL. A panel of cyclic secondary amine-substituted nitrofuranyl amides with the best MIC values was selected for *in vivo* testing. The results were disappointed as the compounds showed little efficacy despite being potent *in vitro* [145]. Studies of the bio-availability showed that they have short biological half-lives and were rapidly eliminated or degraded. Benzylic amide and benzylpiperazine bonds were found at the sites of possible rapid metabolic cleavage.

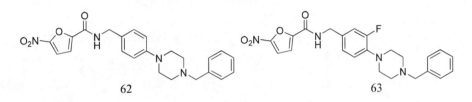

62   63

To develop the third generation, a group of carbamates was prepared. The biological evaluation showed their excellent anti-tuberculosis activity and better solubility. The most active were ethylcarbamate (64) with MIC$_{90}$ = 0.0062 µg/mL and cyclic 4,5-dihydrooxazole analogue (65) that has shown a MIC$_{90}$ value even of 0.00005 µg/mL [146].

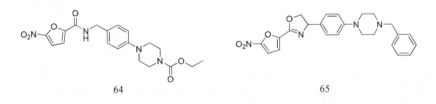

64   65

The amide linkage was thought to be the major reason for the observed metabolic instability. Thus, the replacement of the amide linker with an isoxazoline linker represents a stable bioisosteric replacement for the amide bond. These compounds had better anti-tuberculosis activity *in vitro* and had improved serum half-lives over corresponding compounds in the previous nitrofuranyl amide series [147].

3.2. Targeting P450 Enzymes [148]

The genome of *Mycobacterium tuberculosis* encodes 20 different cytochrome P450 enzymes (P450s), some of which appear to play essential roles. In fungi, these enzymes are the target of azole drugs. The mechanism of their antifungal action includes the inhibition of cytochrome P450 51 (CYP51), which is essential for ergosterol biosynthesis at the step of lanosterol-14-demethylation [149]. Several investigators have tested azoles for anti-tubercular activity [150]. 3-Substituted 5-(pyridin-4-yl)-3H-1,3,4-oxadiazol-2-ones (66; X = substituted heterocycle) can be mentioned as cyclic analogues of INH. These compounds may interact at the active site of the mycobacterial cytochrome P450-dependent sterol 4α-demethylase in the sterol biosynthesis pathway and that their binding free energy values are in agreement with their MIC values (1.25-2.5 µg/mL). 2-Thione derivatives were less active than 2-ones [151].

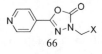

66

P450s are monooxygenases, which are historically considered to facilitate prokaryotic usage of unusual carbon sources. However, their preponderance in *M. tbc.* strongly indicates crucial physiological functions, as does the fact that polycyclic azoles (known P450 inhibitors) have potent anti-mycobacterial effects. Recent structural and enzyme characterization data reveals novel features for at least two *M. tbc.* P450s (CYP121 and CYP51). Genome analysis, knockout studies, and structural comparisons signify important roles in cell biology and pathogenesis for various P450s and redox partner enzymes in *M. tbc.* Elucidation of structure, function, and metabolic roles will be essential in targeting the P450s as an "Achilles heel" in this major human pathogen [152].

3.3. Targeting Isocitrate Lyases

Isocitrate lyase (ICL) is a target enzyme for combatting latent infections of *Mycobacterium tuberculosis*, which is a globally successful pathogen due to its ability to persist for long periods of time unrecognized by the human immune system [153]. The survival of *M. tbc.* in macrophage is the main cause of latent infection. During latency, bacteria are in a slow-growing state and are resistant to the treatment by conventional drugs. To adapt to an inhospitable environment where carbohydrates are limiting and lipids are more abundant in macrophages mycobacteria form glyoxylate cycle. Isocitrate lyase is responsible for the conversion of isocitrate to glyoxylate. This enzyme is absent in mammals. ICL plays a pivotal role in the persistence of *Mycobacterium tuberculosis* in mice by sustaining intracellular infection in inflammatory macrophages [154]. The enzyme allows net carbon gain by diverting acetyl-CoA from beta-oxidation of fatty acids into the glyoxylate shunt pathway. Given its potential as a drug target against persistent infections, its structure was solved without ligand and in complex with two inhibitors. Covalent modification of an active site residue, Cys 191, by the inhibitor 3-bromopyruvate traps the enzyme in a catalytic conformation with the active site completely inaccessible to solvent. The structure of a C191S mutant of the enzyme with the inhibitor 3-nitropropionate provides further insight into the reaction mechanism [155]. The prototype inhibitor of isocitrate lyases is 3-nitropropionic acid [156]. Other compounds that inhibit this enzyme are 3-bromo-2-oxopropionic acid, aconitate, or its derivatives [157].

A role for isocitrate lyase for survival of *Mycobacterium tuberculosis* within macrophage was suggested by the finding that disruption of the *icl* gene inhibited the persistence of mycobacteria in the macrophage. ICL is one of the key enzymes of the glyoxylate metabolism shunt. During the growth on C2 substrates, such as fatty acids or acetate, most microorganisms employ the glyoxylate shunt as the main metabolic route for the biosynthesis of cellular materials. Biochemical studies suggested that in chronically-infected lung tissue, fatty acids might be a major source of carbon for *M. tbc.* Therefore, the failure of the metabolism of fatty acids might partly define the survival failure of the ICL mutant *M. tbc.* in the macrophage and mice. However, primacy of fatty acid metabolism does not rule out the possibility that *M. tbc.* might employ other pathways for carbon metabolism [158]. Since human beings have no functional glyoxylate shunt, the ICL protein will serve as a promising drug target.

3.4. FtsZ-Targeting Compounds

Filamentation temperature-sensitive protein Z (FtsZ) is an essential cell division protein in bacteria and has been shown to be a homologue of the mammalian cytoskeletal protein tubulin. FtsZ is involved in the Z-ring formation and initiation of cell division [159]. In the presence of GTP, FtsZ polymerization is initiated at a single site on the inner membrane at mid-cell and appears to grow bi-directionally to form a highly dynamic helical structure, designated as the Z-ring that encircles the cell. Assembly of the FtsZ is regulated by the FtsZ-interacting proteins, which include stabilizing factors, such as ZapA, ZipA, and FtsA, as well as destabilizing factors, such as SulA, EzrA, and MinCD. Hence, the stability of FtsZ is precisely tuned. Inactivation of FtsZ results in a complete absence of septum formation. The Z-ring is extremely dynamic, continuously remodelling itself. Understanding the FtsZ polymer dynamics will aid in the development of drugs that can prevent cell division by disrupting Z-ring formation. Accordingly, FtsZ is a very promising target for new antimicrobial drug development because of its central role in the cell division and its own biochemical activity. Compounds targeting *M. tbc.* FtsZ were thiabendazole and albendazole. They delay the *M. tbc.* cell division process at MIC 16 μg/mL [160].

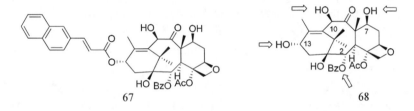

67   68

Taxanes represent such a group of compounds acting on the FtsZ. They exhibit two diverse groups: highly cytotoxic taxoids (*i.e.* "taxol-like compounds") and non-cytotoxic taxane-multidrug resistance agents, which exhibited significant anti-TB activity. Compound *SB-RA-2001* (67) [161] bearing a (*E*)-3-(naphthalen-2-yl)acryloyl group at C-13 position was sensitive with MIC_{99} 2.5-5 μM and was selected as the lead compound for further optimization. A new library of taxanes was prepared by modification of various positions in the molecule of 10-deacetylbaccatin III (DAB; 68).

Four other highly promising noncytotoxic taxanes derived from C-*seco*-baccatin, SB-RA-5001 (69), SB-RA-5001MeO6 (70), SB-RA-50011 (71), and SB-RA-5012 (72) were prepared and possessed potent anti-TB activity (MIC 1.15-2.5 μM) against drug-sensitive and drug-resistant *M. tbc.* strains without appreciable cytotoxicity (IC_{50} > 80 μM) [162].

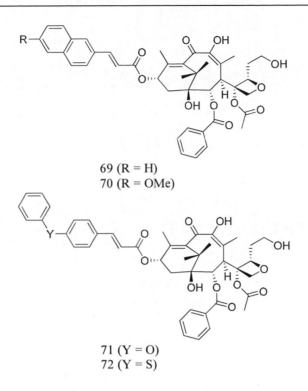

69 (R = H)
70 (R = OMe)

71 (Y = O)
72 (Y = S)

2-Alkoxycarbonylaminopyridines were developed as inhibitors of tubulin polymerization. They inhibit also growth of *M. tbc.* The most active compound *SRI-3072*, ethyl 8-[5-(diethylamino)-4-methylpentan-2-ylamino]-2,3-diphenyl-pyrido[2,3-*b*]pyrazin-6-ylcarbamate (73), exhibited MIC 0.15 μg/mL; it reduced also the growth of *M. tbc.* in mouse-derived macrophages and was specific for FtsZ and did not affect the polymerization of tubulin [163].

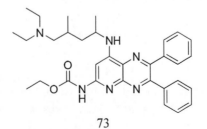

73

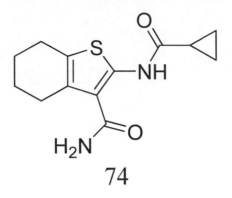

74

3.6. Other Targets

Inhibition of bacterial kinases [164]

The *M. tbc.* genome encodes some proteins, especially protein kinases that act on and intervene in host cell signalling pathways. The mycobacterial serine/threonine protein kinases, PknA, PknB, and PknG, play a key role in keeping the phagosomes intact within the macrophages. It has been demonstrated that the inhibition of PknG leads to the degradation of the mycobacteria by inducing lysosomal-phagosomal fusion [165]. Protein kinase PknG is secreted by pathogenic mycobacteria, in macrophages to intervene with host cell signalling pathways and to block the fusion of the lysosomes with the phagosome by a still unknown mechanism. Compound *AX20017*, 2-(cyclopropanecarboxamido)-4,5,6,7-tetrahydrobenzo[*b*]thiophene-3-carbox-amide (74), from the class of the tetrahydrobenzothiophenes was developed as a lead molecule with IC_{50} values in the nanomolar range, and demonstrated its anti-tuberculotic effects on human macrophages. It might serve the purpose of inducing phagosomal-lysosomal fusion and therefore destroy the residence of the intracellular mycobacteria. It is unclear at this time if these "homeless" mycobacteria are being killed by the host, but they will be at least vulnerable to the activity of anti-mycobacterial agents [166].

Gyrase Blockers

Many potent anti-mycobacterial acting groups could be notionally-derived from quinolones, e.g. 2-substituted derivatives of 3-nitro-5,12-dihydro-5-oxobenzothiazolo[3,2-*a*]-1,8-naphthyridine-6-carboxylic acid. A tested MDR-TB strain was resistant to INH, RIF, EMB, and ofloxacin

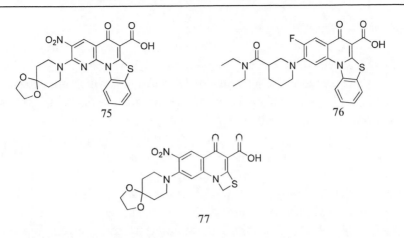

75   76

77

2-(1,4-Dioxa-8-azaspiro[4.5]dec-8-yl)-3-nitro-5,12-dihydro-5-oxobenzo
thiazolo-[3,2-*a*]-1,8-naphthyridine-6-carboxylic acid (75) was found as the
most active compound *in vitro* with MIC = 0.04 μM for this resistant
Mycobacterium tuberculosis. All members of this group showed good activity
and low cytotoxicity. Comparison of activities of the substituents in position 2
took knowledge that most active are substituted piperidines [167]. Similar to
this structure is an anti-mycobacterial acting compound with fluoro
substitution in position 3 instead nitro group and with isosteric substitution of
pyrimidine by benzene, too. The most active from the fluoro substituted
compounds is 2-[3-(diethylcarbamoyl)piperidin-1-yl]-3-fluoro-5,12-dihydro-
5-oxobenzothiazolo[3,2-*a*]quinoline-6-carboxylic acid (76); its MIC on MDR-
TB is 0.08 μM. These benzothiazoloquinolone derivatives were tested for their
ability to inhibit the supercoiling activity of DNA gyrase, like
fluoroquinolones, with the result that tested compounds inhibit *M. smegmatis*
DNA gyrase [168]. Other quinolones-derived derivatives with anti-
mycobacterial activity are 6-fluoro (or 6-nitro)-4-oxo-7-(substituent)-4*H*-
[1,3]thiazeto[3,2-*a*]quinoline-3-carboxylic acids. The most active 7-(1,4-
dioxa-8-azaspiro[4.5]dec-8-yl)-6-nitro-4-oxo-4*H*-[1,3]thiazeto[3,2-
a]quinoline-3-carboxylic acid (77) has MIC lower than 0.09 μM against *M.
tbc*. (H_{37}Rv) and MDR-TB. Compounds with 6-nitro group demonstrated
higher activity then 6-fluoro substitution and for substitution in position 7 are
conveniently-fused piperazines, piperidines, and pyrrolidines [169].

Inhibition of Efflux Pumps

It was described that agents inhibiting efflux pumps of drug-resistant bacteria and cancer cells enhance the killing of intracellular mycobacteria, possibly by increasing the availability of K^+ and Ca^{2+}, which are needed for the activation of lysosomal enzymes of the phagolysosomal unit. Because *organosilicon* compounds (SILA) have recently been demonstrated to inhibit MDR efflux pumps of cancer cells and to reverse the multidrug-resistance of *E. coli*, newly synthesized compounds SILA 409 (78) and SILA 421 (79) were tested for *in vitro* and *ex vivo* activity against XDR-TB. This study investigated the efficacy on *Mycobacterium tuberculosis* strain $H_{37}Rv$ (susceptible to first-line anti-tuberculotics) and clinical isolate resistant to INH, RIF, STR, EMB, PZA, amikacin, kanamycin, capreomycin, ofloxacin, cycloserine, and *p*-aminosalicylic acid (XDR-TB). The activity of the SILA compounds against the susceptible and the XDR-TB strains was identical – SILA 409 exhibiting MIC of 12.5 μg/mL, SILA 421 of 3.125 μg/mL. *Ex vivo* activity of these compounds against phagocytized XDR-TB was evaluated at 0.1 μg/mL. SILA 421 was able to enhance the killing of intracellular mycobacteria by the human macrophage, whereas SILA 409 was inactive. Generally, SILA 421 was shown to have *in vitro* activity against XDR-TB and to transform non-killing macrophages into effective killers of phagocytized bacteria, without any cytotoxic activity. SILA 421 has the potential to be used as a helper compound in the treatment of MDR/XDR-TB infections with a significant *in vitro* anti-tuberculous activity (MIC < 3.5 μg/mL) [170].

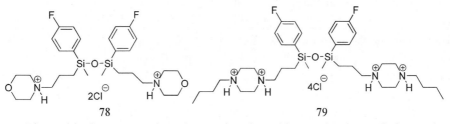

78   79

Phenothiazines are other drugs showing this mechanism of the action [171] (see chapter 3.6.).

Shikimate Pathway

Another possible target for treatment of tuberculosis is the mycobacterial shikimate pathway. It has been shown that this pathway is essential for the viability of *M. tbc.* because it is necessary for the biosynthesis of precursors of aromatic compounds including aromatic amino acids, naphthoquinones and ubiquinones, menaquinones, mycobactin, and other compounds, e.g. folic acid. Additionally, this enzymatic system is absent in human cells which is why the enzymes of this pathway can be promising targets for the development of nontoxic anti-mycobacterial agents. The converted 3-deoxy-D-arabino-heptulosonate-7-phosphate to chorismate in the shikimate biosynthetic pathway of *M. tbc.* Shikimate kinase is the fifth enzyme in the shikimate pathway that catalyzes the phosphate transfer from ATP to shikimate and generates shikimate 3-phosphate and ADP. Some inhibitors of this enzyme were studied, e.g. structural analogues and derivatives of triazole and tetrazole [172,173].

Siderophore Biosynthesis

Inhibition of siderophore biosynthesis may be a potent facility of targeting *M. tuberculosis*. A series was evaluated of 2-triazole derivatives of 5'-[N-(2-hydroxybenzoyl)sulfamoyl]adenosine (80), which inhibits aryl acid-adenylating enzymes involved in siderophore biosynthesis. Compounds with 2- and 4-aminophenyl and pyridin-2/3/4-yl substituents on triazole ring were found as the most potent. *M. tuberculosis* synthesizes structurally aryl-capped siderophores (mycobactines; general structure 81), whereas aryl acid adenylation enzymes perform the installation of the aryl moiety during the biosynthesis of the siderophores. It is probably that siderophores are necessary for virulence, and, additionally, are not present in human organisms [174].

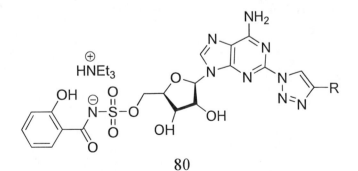

80

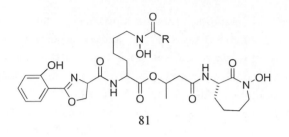

81

Biotin Biosynthesis

The biosynthesis of biotin (vitamin H), a cofactor for carboxylases, decarboxylases, and transcarboxylases, has been identified as an interesting target for antibiotics. This metabolic pathway is specific to microorganisms and higher plants. Diaminopelargonic acid (DAPA) aminotransferase, a pyridoxal 5′-phosphate enzyme involved in biotin biosynthesis, catalyzes the transamination of 8-amino-7-oxononanoic acid using S-adenosyl-L-methionine as an amino donor. This enzyme is present in M. tuberculosis and could be employed as a potential therapeutic target. The naturally-occurring L-amino acid amiclenomycin (82) and its new analogue, 3-[(1s,4s)-4-aminocyclohexa-2,5-dienyl]propan-1-ol (83), were demonstrated to be suicide substrates of this enzyme. The inactivation was irreversible, but a reversal of the antibiotic's effect was observed after the addition of biotin or DAPA. Data indicates that the named alcohol is able to go across the cell wall. The in vivo effect was tested on a wild-type strain of M. smegmatis CIP 56.5. The minimal concentration completely inhibiting the growth in the medium without biotin was 10 µg/mL. A MIC value of amiclenomycin has been reported to range from 3 to 6 µg/mL) [175].

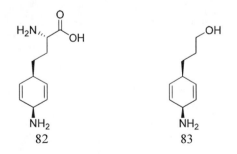

82   83

Other Potential Targets

There are many enzymatic systems in *Mycobacterium tuberculosis* and some of them could be aimed as potential targets for the development of new anti-tuberculous drugs. Nathan et al. [176] referred about such possible targets – the Uvr system liable for macromolecular reparation to maintain DNA integrity during its persistence in the nitrosative and oxidative environment. Proteasomes have the diverse functions including providing a rapid means of adaptation to changing conditions, an irreversible degradation of oxidized or nitrosated proteins, and cannibalizing proteins with low priority to survive amino acids starvation. Two proteasome inhibitors, a peptidyl boronate and epoxomycin, each prevented growth of *M. tbc.* and were mycobactericidal during the recovery of *Mycobacterium tuberculosis* from exposure to reactive nitrogen intermediates. Acids damage macromolecules and interfere with the biochemical reactions and are considered to be a major antimicrobial defence of phagocytes. *M. tbc.* is able to prevent the acidification of phagosomes; however, the activation of macrophages with IFN-γ relieves this block and phagosomes acidify. Nonetheless, *M. tbc.* resists the low pH of this compartment. Strains mutant in a membrane-associated serine protease were hypersensitive to the acidified medium – a deficiency in the membrane protease makes mycobacteria susceptible to the host environment and therefore it represents an attractive drug target. Unlike other bacteria, *M. tuberculosis* possesses a unique defence system that links antioxidant and metabolic pathways. It includes peroxiredoxin, thioredoxin-like protein, dihydrolipoamide acyltransferase, and lipoamide dehydrogenase. These enzymes execute together function as an NADH-dependent peroxynitrite reductase and peroxidase. Dihydrolipoamide transferase mutant *M. tbc.* replicated poorly *in vitro*, was more susceptible to nitrosative stress, and showed lower persistence then wild-types and was described as essential for pathogenesis in a guinea pig model of tuberculosis. Rhodanines are inhibitors of thioredoxin-like proteins and dihydrolipoamide acyltransferase, non-toxic to mammalian cells and bactericidal to *M. bovis* BCG and *M. tbc.* H$_{37}$Rv *in vivo* and *in vitro* and they demonstrated that they could selectively kill non-replicating bacteria. Because lipoamide dehydrogenase is the only functional lipoamide dehydrogenase in *M. tbc.*, targeting or disrupting of this enzyme may result in a more severe phenotype than targeting or disrupting of dihydrolipoamide transferase. Further targets in intermediary metabolism could be other ketoacid dehydrogenases and decarboxylases.

Rhodanine derivatives were described to inhibit the mycobacterial cell wall biosynthesis. They affect four enzymes that form dTDP-rhamnose from dTTP and glucose-1-phosphate [177]. Thus, an essential rhamnose biosynthetic pathway is another perspective target. It is inhibited by 2,3,5-trisubstituted-thiazolidin-4-ones, which docked into the active site cavity of 6'-hydroxyl; dTDP-6-deoxy-D-xylo-4-hexulose 3,5-epimerase from *M. tubercu-losis*. Some of the new compound showed 50% inhibitory activity (at 20 μM) in the coupled rhamnose synthetic assay and some few had modest activity against whole-cell *M. tuberculosis* [178].

4. INVESTIGATION OF "NON-ANTI-TUBERCULOUS" DRUGS AND THEIR DERIVATIVES

One of the possible approaches to discover anti-mycobacterial agents is the investigation of known both antibiotic and non-antibiotic substances. For example, beta-lactams have not been regarded as useful drugs for the treatment of tuberculosis because *M. tbc.* is naturally resistant to most of these antibiotics *in vitro*. This mechanism of resistance is based on the hydrolyzing of penicillins and cephalosporins by beta-lactamase. The resistance may be overcome by the inhibition of the beta-lactamase and by using an antibiotic, which is not a substrate for it. An example of the first way is the use of the combination of *amoxicillin* with a beta-lactamase inhibitor *clavulanate*, which is active *in vitro* and has early bactericidal activity in patients with pulmonary tuberculosis. Anecdotal, amoxicillin-clavulanate in combination with other second-line drugs has been successfully used in selected patients infected with MDR-TB. This approach has met considerable scepticism, and the role of amoxicillin-clavulanate is still unclear. *Imipenem* and *meropenem*, two derivatives of carbapenem, offer a second approach and they are active *in vitro* against *M. tuberculosis*. The efficacy of imipenem was investigated except in a mouse model of tuberculosis in ten patients with MDR-TB (from five- to ten-drug-resistant strains) in the combination with other first- or second-line anti-tuberculotics. Eight of ten patients with numerous risk factors for poor outcomes responded to an imipenem combination therapy with a conversion of cultures to negative. Seven of them remained culture-negative after termination of the treatment without any relapses. There were two deaths, one of which was due to active tuberculosis. Relapse upon withdrawal of imipenem and development of resistance to imipenem in a non-responder suggests that imipenem exerts anti-mycobacterial activity in humans infected with *M. tuberculosis* [179].

　　Macrolides include erythromycin, clarithromycin, azithromycin, and other clinically-used compounds. The first and second-generation macrolides exhibit a weak anti-TB activity although they are very active against the *Mycobacterium avium complex*, Modification of the third generation drugs (telithromycin; 84) has shown activity against *M. tbc.* [180].

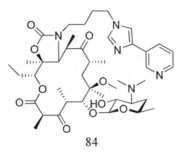

84

　　Some of new macrolide derivatives were investigated because of their activity against drug-resistant isolates of *M. tuberculosis*. This new macrolide RU-66252 (85), RU-69874 (86) and RU-60887 (87) has shown lower MIC on MDR-TB strains than clarithromycin. The most active RU-66252 is a 11,12-carbazate macrolide, RU-69874 is an 11,12-carbamate derivative, RU-60887 is an 11,12-diol derivative of erythromycin. Their MIC on RIF- and INH- (and EMB or STM, in addition) resistant strains of *M. tbc.* range from 0.5 to 4.0 μM. This class is also promising for clinical use for treatment of tuberculosis [181].

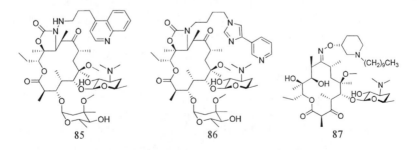

85　　　　　　　　　　86　　　　　　　　　　87

　　Another well-known drug, non-steroidal anti-inflammatory agent *diclofenac* (as a sodium salt), has shown remarkable inhibitory activity on both drug-sensitive and drug-resistant clinical isolates of various Gram-positive, Gram-negative bacteria, and mycobacteria. MIC of diclofenac against tested 45 strains of various mycobacteria ranged from 10 to 25 µg/mL (MIC for 50% of the organisms = 20 µg/mL). 18 strains were sensitive to first-line anti-tuberculotics, 8 were multidrug-resistant, and 19 were polydrug-resistant. MIC of diclofenac is five to six times higher than that of conventional drugs. Even multidrug-resistant clinical strains were susceptible to diclofenac, although some at a higher concentration (25 µg/mL). Diclofenac used in combination with streptomycin augments synergically its efficacy *in vitro* and in murine tuberculosis model. A diclofenac dose of 10 mg/kg/day or 150 mg/kg/day of STM for 4 weeks significantly lowered bacterial counts and reduced the mean spleen weight of mice compared with untreated animals, whereas the simultaneous administration of both agents further decreased CFU counts in the lungs and spleen compared with mice receiving STM alone. In addition, the diclofenac enhanced the antibacterial effect of gentamicin and ceftriaxone, but its anti-inflammatory properties did not appear to affect therapeutic efficacy. The antibacterial activity of diclofenac was found being due to the inhibition of bacterial DNA synthesis; therefore, the compounds could show a wide spectrum of antibacterial, antiprotozoal, antiviral, and antitumor activities. Diclofenac may afford significant protection (at a dose of 10 mg/kg body weight) to mice challenged with virulent *M. tuberculosis* and it is a known immunoregulator and has been shown to up-regulate inflammatory cytokines such as TNF, INF-γ, and IL-2 in *M. tbc.* infection, possibly due to its inhibition of prostaglandins synthesis [182].

Methyl-L-DOPA has been used as antihypertensive agent for many years. It was discovered that it has significant *in vitro* activity against atypical mycobacteria (*M. avium complex, M. scrofulaceum, M. xenopi, M. marinum, and M. fortuitum*). It was assayed for its *in vitro* activity against 53 different strains of mycobacteria, including 34 clinical isolates of both drug-sensitive and drug-resistant *M. tuberculosis*. Most of the strains were inhibited at 10-25 µg/mL concentrations of the drug. After an injection of methyl-L-DOPA into male mice at a concentration of 10 mg/kg body weight (20 g each), methyl-L-DOPA significantly protected them when challenged with a 50 median lethal dose of *M. tuberculosis* [183].

Phenothiazines are widely used drugs, namely in psychiatry as antipsychotic agents due to a blockade, especially of dopamine receptors. Their antibacterial activity was described in 1959. More recently, chlorpromazine has been shown to inhibit the growth of *M. tuberculosis* ingested by macrophages. Although this action is achieved by concentrations of chlorpromazine used for treatment of psychoses (0.5-1.0 µg/mL), the adverse neurological effects often encountered at such concentrations would prevent any practical applications of chlorpromazine for the management of tuberculosis. The anti-mycobacterial action of phenothiazines is independent of the neuroleptic activity. MIC of chlorpromazine and thioridazine on both INH- and RIF-resistant clinical isolated strains (and with other facultative resistance to one or more drugs of PZA, EMB, and STM ranged from 8 to 32 µg/mL. Additionally, chlorpromazine significantly inhibited the generation of $^{14}CO_2$ at concentration of 2 µg/mL [184]. Other source cites the lowest effective concentration of chlorpromazine for INH-, RIF-, STR-, and EMB-resistant strains 4 µg/mL, of thioridazine 2 µg/mL and for drug-susceptible strains 2 µg/mL (both compounds). The other phenothiazines with reported anti-mycobacterial activity are e.g. levomepromazine, trifluoperazine, and methdilazine [185].

The order of the activity against MDR-TB of four phenothiazines was chlorpromazine = thioridazine > promethazine > promazine. The levels required for an MIC_{50} exceeded 1 µg/mL and are beyond those that are clinically achievable, but phenothiazines are concentrated in macrophages that phagocytose and have *in situ* activity against mycobacteria. These agents may be considered for use as adjuvant for the management of freshly diagnosed tuberculosis in patients from populations with a high prevalence of MDR-TB, at least for the interval during which the antibiotic susceptibility of the isolate is being determined [186]. When the prognosis is poor, available therapy is ineffective and death is inevitable; compassionate therapy with thioridazine should be contemplated because the risks are small and the rewards could be great [187]. As this period would be only a few months, side effects associated with the neuroleptics are not anticipated. Chlorpromazine, which produces severe and frequent side effects, had the same average activity as the "mild" neuroleptic thioridazine [186].

Phenothiazines affect a number of mycobacterial targets. It was described that phenothiazines do transform non-killing macrophages into effective killers. It seems possible that this killing is enhanced by the phenothiazine's inhibition of the K^+ efflux from the phagolysosome dependent upon Ca^{2+}-dependent ATPase. They also inhibit the binding of calcium to calmodulin of mammalian cells and to calmodulin-like proteins of bacteria. The inhibition of calcium access to Ca^{2+}-dependent ATPase inhibits transport processes such as those performed by influx and efflux pumps. Bacteria, as well as mammalians, contain efflux pumps that extrude toxic agents from the periplasm and cytoplasm of the former and from the cytoplasm of the latter. Phenothiazines readily intercalate between nucleic bases of the DNA helix and the degree of intercalation is dependent upon the number of guanosine-cytosine residues. When phenothiazines intercalate into DNA, they inhibit all DNA-based processes as well as the degree of the coiling and the uncoiling of DNA promoted by the gyrases. The inhibition of the efflux pump by a phenothiazine would result in large numbers of phenothiazine molecules entering the cell, reaching the DNA, and thereby inhibiting the replication of the bacterium [171]. Development of resistance to phenothiazines is unlikely, as mutations affecting the mycobacterial calcium flux would affect the viability of the microorganism [188].

Of particular interest is that trifluoperazine exhibited a significant decreasing effect on *in vitro* ATP synthesis by *M. leprae*. Genomic analysis of *Mycobacterium tuberculosis* led to the identification of type II nicotinamide adenine dinucleotide dehydrogenase (NADH) as a key enzyme for bacterial growth under aerobic conditions and a unique and specific target for drug action because in human mitochondria only type I NADH dehydrogenase is present, whereas in mycobacteria both types are present. Based on some experiments, Weinstein et al. [189] affirmed that the anti-tuberculous activity of phenothiazines appears to be partially due to the specific inhibition of type II NADH dehydrogenase, as determined by NADH: menaquinone oxidoreductase activity [188]. It was demonstrated that trifluoperazine binds directly to NADH-2 as a non-competitive inhibitor with respect to NADH and is uncompetitive with respect to the primary quinone substrate, ubiquinone Q2 [190]. The modulation of electron transport in mycobacteria by phenothiazines may have a profound effect on the entrance and maintenance of dormancy [189].

Phenothiazines have been shown to enhance the activity of antibiotics and anti-tuberculotics (except ethambutol) to which bacteria are susceptible. This might result in a reduction in the dose of some or all of the antibiotics. Chlorpromazine, thioridazine, and promethazine were shown to enhance the activity of RIF and STM when used in combinations at concentrations that are minimally effective when employed separately against clinical strains of *M. tuberculosis* resistant to two or more antibiotics (polydrug resistance), but they had no effect on the activity of isoniazid against polydrug-resistant *M. tbc.* strains. These phenothiazines enhanced the activity at concentrations that produce little or no direct activity against these strains. Increased permeability after administration of phenothiazines might enhance the activity of RIF and STM, both acting within the cell, whereas the catalase-peroxidase converting INH to active form might be external to the plasma membrane. However, other authors found chlorpromazine enhanced the activity of isoniazid as well as streptomycin and rifampicin, but there was no increasing in ethambutol activity [191].

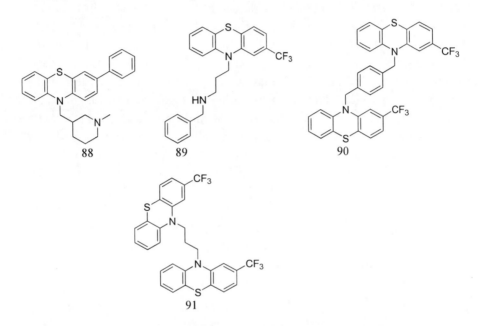

Some analogues of phenothiazine were synthesized and examined as antitubercular agents against *M. tuberculosis* $H_{37}Rv$. The compounds were subsequently screened for binding to the dopaminergic-receptor subtypes D_1, D_2, D_3, and the serotonergic-receptor subtypes $5-HT_{1A}$, $5-HT_{2A}$, and $5-HT_{2C}$. These receptors are primarily responsible for the psychotropic effects. The most active compounds showed MIC from 2 to 4 µg/mL and had an overall reduced binding to the dopamine and serotonin receptors in comparison to chlorpromazine and trifluoperazine. The antipsychotic phenothiazine drugs have a basic side chain at the 10-position, the distal nitrogen was maintained and added diverse substitutions with both an alkyl and a benzyl linker. 10-[(1-Methylpiperidin-3-yl)methyl]-3-phenyl-10*H*-phenothiazine (88) was the most potent with MIC (*M. tbc.* $H_{37}Rv$) of 2.1 µg/mL. The increased activity of the phenyl-substituted phenothiazine rings suggests that there may be space for additional steric interaction in the receptor binding pocket in this region. The replacement of the phenothiazine ring with another ring and an introduction of a heteroatom into the ring system led to significant decreasing of the activity. The compounds with substitutions on the side chain generally led to a loss in activity, but N-benzyl-3-[2-(trifluoromethyl)-10H-phenothiazin-10-yl]propan-1-amine (89) showed an MIC of 4.2 μg/mL. In general, the compounds with the benzyl substitution and bulkier side chains were less active. Interestingly, the two bis-phenothiazines were both potent compounds – 1,4-bis{[2-(trifluoromethyl)-10H-phenothiazin-10-yl]methyl}benzene (90) with an MIC 2.3 μg/mL and 1,3-bis[2-(trifluoromethyl)-10H-phenothiazin-10-yl]propane (91) with an MIC 2.0 μg/mL. All these compounds were screened for binding to the named receptors. The ring-substitution analogues retained high binding to most of the receptors with some loss in affinities to the D_1, 5-HT_{1A}, and 5-HT_{2C} receptors and 10-[(1-methylpiperidin-3-yl)methyl]-3-phenyl-10H-phenothiazine had a little tendency to bind to the serotonin receptors, but had only a moderate reduction in affinity for the dopamine receptors. The compounds with an alkyl linker and diversity at the pendant nitrogen retained generally a binding profile similar to that of the control drugs. Overall, presented data indicated that an increase in the steric volume on the side chain reduces binding to these subtypes of the dopamine and serotonin receptors. The two bi-phenothiazine compounds have substantially reduced binding to the dopamine and serotonin receptors [190].

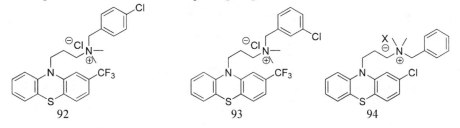

Another approach to reduce the undesirable side effects of phenothiazines is the quarterization of chlorpromazine, triflupromazine, and promethazine derivatives. These compounds were examined against both actively-growing and non-replicating *M. tuberculosis* $H_{37}Rv$ (unfortunately, no data about MDR-TB was presented). Several compounds inhibited non-replicating *M. tbc.* at concentrations equal to or double their MIC against the actively-growing strain. All active compounds did not show toxicity toward Vero cells ($IC_{50} > 128$ μM). It was described that N-benzylchlorpromazinium inhibited

M. tbc. in vitro at an even lower concentration than chlorpromazine itself. *N*-Benzyl substitution in quaternized derivatives is a requirement for significant anti-tubercular activity; alkyl-chain branching decreases potency and an electron-withdrawing substituent on the phenothiazine ring was also essential. Three of the derivatives having an MIC both < 4 μM against actively growing *M. tbc.* and < 8 μM against non-replicating *M. tbc.* possess *N*-(4- or 3-chlorobenzyl)groups and electron-withdrawing substituents on the phenothiazine ring. An MIC of an actively growing *M. tbc.* of two of the most active derivatives, *N*-(4-chlorobenzyl)-*N*,*N*-dimethyl-3-[2-(trifluoromethyl)-10*H*-phenothiazin-10-yl]propan-1-aminium chloride (92) and *N*-(3-chlorobenzyl)-*N*,*N*-dimethyl-3-[2-(trifluoromethyl)-10*H*-phenothiazin-10-yl]-propan-1-aminium chloride (93), were 3.81 and 3.8 μM, and MIC values of non-replicating mycobacteria were 6.1 and 5.8 μM, respectively [192].

Among newly-prepared phenothiazines, *N*-benzyl-3-(2-chloro-10*H*-phenothiazin-10-yl)-*N*,*N*-dimethylpropan-aminium salt (94) is 12-fold more potent than trifluoperazine, and, in contrast to it, this compound is water-soluble at pH 7.4. Its MIC was determined as 1.11 μg/mL. In mouse model in female BALB/c mice of acute infection by $H_{37}Rv$ *M. tbc.*, a 100 mg/kg dose produced a 1 log decrease in CFU within the lung, and animals treated with this compound showed no CFU in the spleen, whereas three of five animals receiving the vehicle alone had recoverable organisms [189].

Some derivatives of thioridazine were synthesized, patented, and denoted with their own code – therefore their structures are not presented here. All of these derivatives have activity against the *M. tuberculosis* $H_{37}Rv$ and a few (#1867, #1870 and #1875) have similar activity (their MIC are 5, 10, 5 μg/mL, respectively) to that of thioridazine (MIC = 2,5 μg/mL). The toxicity evaluation showed that at concentrations equivalent to that associated with toxicity for thioridazine, no significant toxicity was detected. All of the derivatives at a concentration of 0.1 μg/mL enhanced the killing of intracellular *M. tuberculosis*. Furthermore, in contrast to the killing effect of thioridazine where it takes 3 days to kill all of the phagocytosed *M. tuberculosis*, these compounds killed all of the phagocytosed organisms within 1 day [193].

Benzylamine mucolytics *ambroxole* and *bromhexine* showed a pH-dependent growth-inhibitory effect on clinical isolates of *M. tuberculosis*. Inhibition of mycobacterial growth was more evident at a low pH. These compounds are concentrated in macrophages, and might exert a clinically useful effect on intracellular tubercle bacilli. This combined with indirect effects including enhancement of lysozyme bronchial secretions and rifampicin levels in lung tissue and sputum and possibly clearance of bacilli-laden mucus from cavities and bronchi suggests a potentially useful adjunctive function in the therapy of tuberculosis [194].

5. OTHER ACTIVE SYNTHETIC COMPOUNDS

Some *pyridine* and *purine analogues* were found to be active against *M. tbc*. 9-Benzyl-2-chloro-6-(furan-2-yl)purine (95) exhibited relative low toxicity against mammalian cells and are highly active against drug-resistant strains of *M. tbc*. A thiol analogue of purine, 2-[6-(dodecylthio)-9*H*-purin-9-yl]butanoic acid (96), was also highly active against *M. tbc*. with MIC of 0.78 µg/mL ad SI > 12.8 [195]. Barrow et al. [196] reported that 2-methyladenosine (97) displayed good activity against *M. tbc*. with an MIC of < 1.56-3.12 µg/mL for various strains, including resistant strains and non-replicating *M. tbc*. in an *in vitro* hypoxic shift-down model.

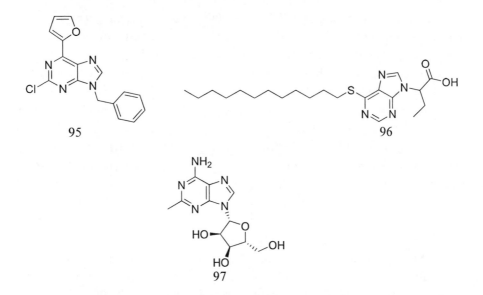

The sulfonamide group is considered as the pharmacophore, which is present in a number of biologically active molecules. 4*H*-1,2,4-Benzothiadiazine 1,1-dioxides can be considered as a cyclic sulfonamide class of molecules containing pyrazine-2-carbohydrazide as a substituent at the 3-

position of 4*H*-1,2,4-benzothiadiazine 1,1-dioxide (98) demonstrated excellent anti-mycobacterial activity with an MIC of 0.5-2.0 µg/mL against both drug-resistant and drug-sensitive clinical isolates of *M. tbc.* (H_{37}Rv ATCC 27294) and an MIC of 2.0 µg/mL against *M. avium* (ATCC 49601) and *M. intracellulare* (ATCC 13950) [197]. A combination of benzothiadiazine-sulphones with nitrofuran led to the preparation of a new series with improved bio availability and good anti-mycobacterial activity. The most active was compound (99) with an MIC of 1 µg/mL against *M. tbc.* [198].

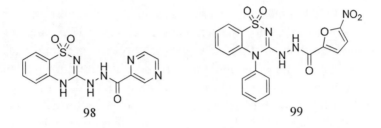

98   99

An efficacy against MDR-TB has been shown by derivatives of 2-amino-6-methyl-4-aryl-8-[(*E*)-arylmethylidene]-5,6,7,8-tetrahydro-4*H*-pyrano[3,2-*c*]pyridine-3-carbonitriles. As the most potent compound was described 2-amino-4-[4-(dimethylamino)phenyl]-8-(*E*)-[4-(dimethylamino)phenyl]-methylidene-6-methyl-5,6,7,8-tetrahydro-4*H*-pyrano[3,2-*c*]-pyridine-3-carbo-nitrile (100). Its MIC on the multidrug-resistant mycobacterial strain (resistant to isoniazid, rifampicin, ethambutol, and ofloxacin) was 0.43 µM. The anti-mycobacterial activity is generally enhanced (the most active compound is an exception) by the presence of weak electron-withdrawing groups (*e.g.* chloro- and fluoro-) in the aromatic rings; replacement of phenyl by other heterocyclic rings reduces the activity markedly [199].

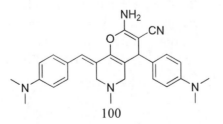

100

Another nitrogen heterocycle is quinoxaline. Its derivatives, ketones and amides of *quinoxaline 1,4-di-N-oxides*, were synthesized and evaluated *in vitro* against *M. tuberculosis* and for efficacy in a murine model of tuberculosis. Tested strains of *M. tbc.* were drug-susceptible $H_{37}Rv$, single-drug-resistant (isoniazid, rifampicin, thioacetazone, ethambutol, *p*-aminosalicylic acid, kanamycin, ethionamide, and ciprofloxacin, and MDR-TB clinical isolates (RIF, INH, and some of them additional resistant to STM, PZA, ETH, or quinolones). The most active compound, 3-acetyl-6-chloro-2-methylquinoxaline 1,4-dioxide (101), showed good activity on drug-susceptible (MIC 0.78 µg/mL), all single-drug-resistant (MIC from 0.39 to 1.56 µg/mL), and MDR strains (0.625 or 1.25 µg/mL). This compound is likely activated via bio-reduction in bacteria, similar to the reduction observed for other substituted *N*-oxides and was chosen for the *in vivo* assessment. It was demonstrated that it showed equal activity on growing and non-replicating bacteria, perhaps because the sterilization shortens the treatment of TB. Preliminary an *in vivo* evaluation was realized with a dose of 300 mg/kg in infected GKO C57BL/6 mice. This compound afforded significant reductions of 2.7 and 2.82 log CFU in the lung and spleen tissues, respectively, in comparison with untreated controls. The compound has a bactericidal effect *in vivo*. Preliminary studies indicate that cytotoxicity and *in vivo* toxicity can be separated from the anti-tubercular activity, although a relatively high dose was used [200]. Quinoxaline derivatives have been further studied; thus, quinoxaline-2-carboxylate 1,4-di-*N*-oxide derivatives were tested *in vitro* against a broad spectrum of single-drug-resistant *M. tuberculosis* with good activity. Very efficacious ethyl 7-chloro-3-methylquinoxaline-2-carboxylate 1,4-dioxide (102) was found during the evaluation in a series of *in vivo* assays to be active in reducing CFU counts in both the lungs and spleens of infected mice by oral administration, efficacious against PA-824-resistant *M. bovis* and very active against non-replicating bacteria adapted to low-oxygen conditions [201]. Another newly prepared group, benzyl quinoxaline-2-carboxylate 1,4-dioxides (103), showed a low MIC (up 0.10 µg/mL) and good efficacy in a *in vitro* TB-infected macrophage model, too, and 6,7-dichloroderivative were evaluated against single-drug-resistant tuberculous strains (EMB, INH, RIF, kanamycin, ETH, or thioacetazone) with MIC ≤ 6.25 µg/mL [202].

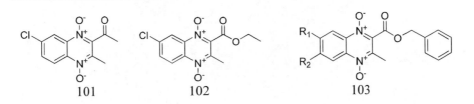

101   102   103

A series of *2-benzylthio derivatives* of *benzoxazole* was synthesized and evaluated against *M. tbc.* and non-tuberculous mycobacteria. Tested MDR strains were resistant to INH, RIF, EMB, STM, ofloxacin, rifabutin, and ciprofloxacin or to INH, RIF, EMB, STM, ofloxacin, and rifabutin or to INH, RIF, gentamicin, amikacin, and rifabutin. The highest activity reached compounds with 3,5-dinitrosubstitution on a phenyl ring – it is probable that this potent anti-mycobacterial activity of 2-(3,5-dinitrobenzylsulfa-nyl)benzoxazole (104) and 2-(2,4-dinitrobenzylsulfanyl)benzoxazole is connected specially with a nitro group. The MIC of 2-(3,5-dinitrobenzyl-sulfanyl)benzoxazole ranged by all named drug-resistant tuberculosis strains from 2 to 4 µM [51].

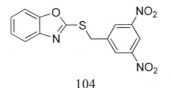

104

A series of novel spiro-pyrido-pyrrolizines and pyrrolidines of *1-methyl-3,5-bis[(E)-arylmethylidene]tetrahydro-4(1H)-pyridinones* were synthesized and screened for anti-mycobacterial activity on *M. tbc.* $H_{37}Rv$ and multidrug-resistant clinical isolated strain *M. tuberculosis* (resistant to isoniazid, rifampicin, ciprofloxacin, and ethambutol) and *M. smegmatis*. Among the prepared compounds, spiro-[2.2″]acenaphthene-1″-one-spiro[3.3′]-5′-(2-chlorophenylmethylidene)-1′-methyltetrahydro-4′(1H)-pyridinone-4-(2-chlorophenyl)hexahydro-1H-pyrrolizine (105) was found to be the most active because the MIC was 0.4 µg/mL against both susceptible and MDR strains [203].

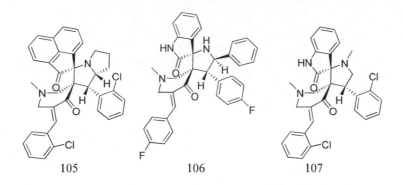

105   106   107

Similar to the preceding series of anti-tuberculotics are *spiro-piperidin-4-ones*. These compounds were evaluated for their *in vitro* and *in vivo* activity against *M. tuberculosis* $H_{37}Rv$, MDR *M. tuberculosis* and *M. smegmatis*. 4-(4-Fluorophenyl)-5-phenylpyrrolo(spiro[2.3″]oxindole)spiro[3.3′]-1′-methyl-5′-(4-fluorophenylmethylidene)piperidin-4′-one (106) was found as the most active with a MIC value of 0.07 µM against drug-susceptible *M. tbc.* and of 0.16 µg/mL against isoniazid-, rifampicin-, ethambutol- and ofloxacin-resistant *M. tbc.* strains, and therefore it is several times more potent than isoniazid and ciprofloxacin. *In vivo* this compound decreased the bacterial load in the lung and spleen tissues with 1.30 and 3.73 log protections, respectively, and was considered to be promising in reducing bacterial count in the lung and spleen. Another compound, 4-(2-chlorophenyl)-1-methylpyrrolo-(spiro[2.3″]oxindole-)-spiro-[3.3′]-1′-methyl-5′-(arylidene)piperidin-4′-one (107), was determined to have an MIC 0.08 µM against MDR-TB and to be 569.6 and 471.6 times more potent than isoniazid and ciprofloxacin, respectively [204].

Various amine derivatives have been known as therapeutic agents. Bacteriostatic activity of tertiary amines, quaternary ammonium salts, and *p*-toluidine moiety have been reported long back and a number of aromatic and heteroaromatic amines were evaluated for their anti-tubercular efficacy and some of them possess very good activity. *N*-Alkyl benzylamines have been reported to be specific anti-tubercular compounds as they are inactive against a number of bacteria and fungi. A series of 42 benzyl- and pyridylmethyl amines were synthesized and evaluated against both avirulent ($H_{37}Ra$) and virulent strains ($H_{37}Rv$) of *M. tuberculosis*. Many of the compounds exhibited an MIC as low as 1.56 µg/mL. Most of these compounds are active in infectious strains ($H_{37}Rv$) only and inactive against avirulent strains ($H_{37}Ra$).

A few of the potent compounds were also evaluated against MDR-TB clinical isolates. The most efficacious compounds (*E*)-[(octadec-9-enylamino)methyl]phenol (108), *N*-(pyridin-4-ylmethyl)hexadecan-1-amine (109; R = pyridin-4-yl) and *N*-(pyridin-3-ylmethyl)hexadecan-1-amine (109; R = pyridin-3-yl) were active at the concentration of MIC = 3.12 μg/mL [205].

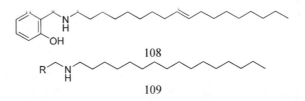

108

109

It was identified that a glycosylated phenyl cyclopropyl methanone (110) showed very good efficacy against MDR strains of *M. tuberculosis* and *in vivo*, too. The cyclopropyl ring is a structural element of the mycobacterial cell wall and its importance in the structures of chemotherapeutics is also well known. Based on the knowledge it was synthesized and evaluated for anti-mycobacterial activity in a group of aryl cyclopropyl methanones and their derivatives. All these compounds have been detected to be active against *M. tbc.* H$_{37}$Rv *in vitro* and most of them with an MIC ranging from 3.125 to 25 μg/mL. Only a few compounds were active against avirulent strain H$_{37}$Ra. Further, cyclopropyl[4-(4-fluorobenzyloxy)phenyl]methanol (111) was also screened against multidrug-resistant strains and evaluated (not alone) in the murine model. This compound completely inhibited the growth of five MDR-TB clinical isolates (except INH and RIF facultative resistant to EMB) at 6.25 μg/mL. Cytotoxicity was assessed in Vero cell line and based on IC$_{50}$ values selectivity index was found to be 10. After a daily dose of 100 mg/kg this compound produced a 17% enhancement in to the mice survival time compared to control without treatment [206].

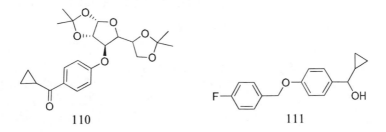

110   111

Thiadiazine thione nucleus has been reported for different biological activities, including tuberculostatic, antibacterial, antiviral, or antifungal. It has been postulated that the biological activity of these molecules is dependent on isothiocyanates and dithiocarbamic acid species generated in the biosystem on hydrolysis. A series of 3,5-disubstituted thiadiazine thiones has been synthesized and screened for anti-tubercular activity *in vitro* against *M. tuberculosis* $H_{37}Rv$. Three compounds presented their activity with an MIC of 12.5 μg/mL. The *in vitro* high MIC values in this series did not discourage because it is known that *in vitro* activity often displays poor correlation with activity *in vivo*, and the reason for this failure is most often conflicting balances between bio-availability and activity. Compounds with thiocarbonyl and sulphide moiety are known to be bio-activated by *S*-oxidation to sulphoxides and sulphones. MIC of the sulphides is much less *in vitro* in comparison to sulphone. 3-(5-Cyclopropyl-6-thioxo-1,3,5-thiadiazinan-3-yl)propanoic acid (112) was tested *in vitro* against five MDR clinical isolates (resistant to INH, RIF, and either ofloxacin and ethambutol or ethambutol or alone) and it exhibited tuberculostatic activity of four of these strains in concentration of 50 μg/mL, too. The mean survival time of the treated mice (100 mg/kg daily) was enhanced; 33% mice were surviving in treated group and the load of bacilli in the lung was considerably less than in the untreated control group [207].

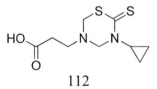

112

6. OTHER ACTIVE, NATURALLY-OCCURRING COMPOUNDS

Natural products represent an alternative in search of new compounds. Marine organisms are rich on various unusual structures. Aerothionin (113) and calafianin (114) isolated from the marine sponge *Aplysina gerardogreeni* were evaluated against multidrug-resistant clinical isolates of *M. tuberculosis*. Aerothionin was also tested against these eight strains with different drug-resistance patterns and nine non-tuberculous mycobacteria species. It was active against all the drug-resistant clinical isolates, regardless of their resistance patterns, with minimum inhibitory concentrations from 6.5 to 25 µg/mL. Three out of nine non-tuberculosis mycobacteria were inhibited by aerothionin: *M. kansasii* (50 µg/mL), *M. scrofulaceum* (100 µg/mL) and *M. avium* (100 µg/mL) [208].

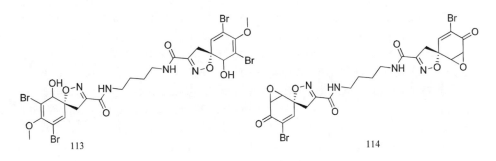

Originally, a group of antibacterial and anti-mycobacterial compounds, β-triketones, was obtained from the natural source, New Zealand´s essential oil from shrub *Leptospermum scoparium* and other plants and trees, especially from the family *Myrtaceae*. Synthetic analogues including phloroglucinols were prepared. This group is active not only on *M. tbc.* but on some resistant Gram-positive bacterial strains (e.g. MRSA and VRE) and fungi (*Trichophyton mentagrophytes*). It seems to be probable that the triketones may act by disrupting the cytoplasmic membrane due to their hydrophobicity. The most active derivative was shown to stimulate oxygen consumption by resting cell suspensions and caused a decreasing of intracellular ATP. There are located vitally important systems in the cytoplasmatic membrane – electron transport chain or ATP synthase complex. It is a reason why these compounds are non-selective only on microbial cells. The tested strain was a clinical isolate (IMCJ945) resistant to isoniazid, rifampicin, ethambutol, streptomycin, kanamycin, ethionamide, and *p*-aminosalicylic acid. The MIC of the most active derivative 4-dodecanoyl-5-hydroxy-2,2,6,6-tetramethyl cyclohex-4-ene-1,3-dione (115) was 2 µg/mL [209].

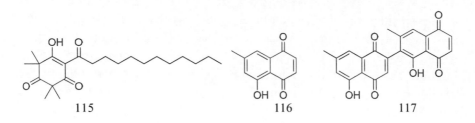

115   116   117

Naphthoquinones and triterpenes were isolated from the roots of the African tree *Euclea natalensis*. One of this compound, 7-methyljuglone (5-hydroxy-7-methylnaphtalene-1,4-dione; 116), was active both to the drug-sensitive and drug-resistant strains of *M. tuberculosis*; MIC ranged from 0.32 to 1.25 µg/mL. Additionally, 7-methyljuglone presented a superior intracellular inhibition of *M. tbc.* in macrophages than in streptomycin and ethambutol [210]. Diospyrin (117), the dimer of 7-methyljuglone, showed activity against drug-sensitive and drug-resistant mycobacterial strains, too [211]. Combinations of 7-methyljuglone with INH and RIF has a synergistic effect and led to multiple reduction of MIC. Thus, 7-methyljuglone can be a promising anti-tuberculous agent. Its mechanism of the action may consist in the inhibition of the oxygen consumption of *M. tuberculosis* or may be due to the influence of the mitochondrial functions that cause repression of pyrimidine biosynthesis by the inhibition of dihydroorotate dehydrogenase. This enzyme is essential for *M. tuberculosis* growth [212]. Other naphthoquinones were described as anti-tuberculosis agents, but less active and with lower selectivity index than 7-methyljuglone. Several of these compounds have been shown to operate as subversive substrates with mycothiol disulfide reductase. The absence of a direct correlation between anti-tubercular activity and subversive substrate efficiency with mycothiol disulfide reductase might be a consequence of their non-specific reactivity with multiple biological targets (e.g. other disulfide reductases) [213].

Some reports referred about anti-tuberculous activity of extracts of medical plants, e.g. [214-218] against susceptible, single-drug or multidrug-resistant mycobacterial strains. It is notable that the composition of the extracts and the occurrence and the mutual proportion of present active compounds may be in every other extract different. Therefore we cannot rank these non-standardized plant extracts in the leading of approaches of development new drugs acting against MDR-TB if no active substance in these different extracts is identified and isolated (like 7-methyljuglone or aegicerin).

Chapter 3

CONCLUSION

While tuberculosis is curable, MDR-TB and XDR-TB may be fatal and the cure rates are frustratingly low. For this purpose, it is necessary to accelerate investigations to identify new types of anti-TB drugs acting on novel drug targets. It is essential to develop the active agent that is bactericidal against persistent and dormant organisms of *M. tbc.* that could shorten the treatment course and eliminate the reservoir of latent strains of *M. tbc.* As it is summarized in the review article, the last decade have shown dramatic progress in understanding the biology, intracellular lifestyle, and detailed biochemistry of the mycobacteria. New drug targets have been observed. High-resolution structures of gene products encoded by virulence genes are available and bioinformatic-based approaches are promising strategies in the fight against MDR-TB. Some promising agents (PA-824, OPC-67683, and TMC207) will be approved for clinical use, although there are some difficulties (*i.e.* mutagenicity, bioavailability, and drug interaction) that should be resolved before their approval.

ACKNOWLEDGMENTS

This work was supported by MSM 0021620822 and IGA NS 10367-3.

REFERENCES

[1]   Wright, A; Zignol, M. Anti-tuberculosis drug resistance in the world (fourth global report) [online]. 2008 [cited 2008-12-6]. Available from: http://www.who.int/tb/publications/2008/drs_report4_26feb08.pdf.

[2]   Zager, EM; McNerney, R. Multidrug-resistant tuberculosis. *BMC Infect. Dis.*, 2008, 8, Article Number 10.

[3]   Jain, A; Dixit, P. Multidrug resistant to extensively drug resistant tuberculosis: What is next? *J. Biosci.*, 2008, 33, 605-616.

[4]   Dye, C; Floyd, K; Gunneberg, C; Hosseini, M; Lonnroth, K; Nathanson, E; Pantoky, A; Piatek, M; Uplekar, M; Watt, C; Williams, B; Wright, A; Zignol, M. Global tuberculosis control: Surveillance, planning, financing: WHO report 2007. 1st ed. Geneva: World Health Organization; 2007.

[5]   Tuberculosis facts 2008 [online]. 2008 [cited 2009-02-09]. Available from: http://www.who.int/tb/publications/2008/factsheet_april08.pdf.

[6]   http://www.tibotec.com/bgdisplay.jhtml?itemname=TB_disease

[7]   Laughon, BE. New tuberculosis drugs in development. *Curr. Top. Med. Chem.*, 2007, 7, 463-473.

[8]   Blanc, L; Chaulet, P; Espinal, M; Graham, S; Grzemska, M; Harries, A; Luelmo, F; Maher, D; O'Brien, R; Raviglione, M; Rieder, H; Starke, J; Uplekar, M; Wells, C. Treatment of tuberculosis guidelines for national programmes [online]. 2008 [cited 2008-12-06]. Available from: http://whqlibdoc.who.int/hq/2003/WHO_CDS_TB_2003.313_eng.pdf.

[9]   Palomino, JC; Leao, SC; Ritacco, V. Tuberculosis 2007: From basic science to patient care [online]. 2007 [cited 2008-12-18]. Available from: http://www.tuberculosistextbook.com/tuberculosis2007.pdf.

[10] Frequently asked questions – XDR-TB [online]. 2006 [cited 2009-02-11]. Available from: http://www.who.int/tb/challenges/xdr/faqs/en/index.html.

[11] Jain, A; Mondal, R. Extensively drug-resistant tuberculosis: Current challenges and threats. *FEMS Immunol. Med. Microbiol.*, 2008, 53, 145-150.

[12] Rich, M (ed.). Guidelines for the programmatic management of drug-resistant tuberculosis [online]. 2008 [cited 2009-02-08]. Available from: http://whqlibdoc.who.int/publications/2008/9789241547581_eng.pdf.

[13] Bardou, F; Raynaud, C; Ramos, C; Laneelle, MA; Laneelle, G. Mechanism of isoniazid uptake in *Mycobacterium tuberculosis*. *Microbiology (UK)*, 1998, 144, 2539-2544.

[14] Shi, R; Itagaki, N; Sugawara, I. Overview of anti-tuberculosis (TB) drugs and their resistance mechanisms. *Mini Rev. Med. Chem.*, 2007, 7, 1177-1185.

[15] Brindley, DN; Matsumur, S; Bloch, K. *Mycobacterium phlei* fatty acid synthetase – a bacterial multienzyme complex. *Nature*, 1969, 224, 666-669.

[16] Vilcheze, C; Morbidoni, HR; Weisbrod, TR; Iwamoto, H; Kuo, M; Sacchettini JC; Jacobs, WR. Inactivation of the inhA-encoded fatty acid synthase II (FAS II) enoyl-acyl carrier protein reductase induces accumulation of the FAS I end products and cell lysis of *Mycobacterium smegmatis*. *J. Bacteriol.*, 2000, 182, 4059-4067.

[17] Petrini, B; Hoffner, S. Drug-resistant and multidrug-resistant tubercle bacilli. *Int. J. Antimicrob. Agents*, 1999, 13, 93-97.

[18] Ramaswamy, SV; Reich, R; Dou, SJ; Jasperse, L; Pan, X; Wanger, A; Quitugua, T; Graviss, EA. Single nucleotide polymorphism in genes associated with isoniazid resistance in *Mycobacterium tuberculosis*. *Antimicrob. Agents Chemother.*, 2003, 47, 1241-1250.

[19] Heym, B; Zhang, Y; Poulet, S; Young, D; Cole, ST. Characterization of the katG gene encoding a catalyse-peroxidase required for the isoniazid susceptibility of *Mycobacterium tuberculosis*. *J. Bacteriol.*, 1993, 175, 4255-4259.

[20] Sander, P; Böttger, EC. Mycobacteria: Genetics of resistance and implications for treatment. *Chemotherapy*, 1999, 45, 95-108.

[21] Cohen, T; Becerra, MC; Murray, MB. Isoniazid resistance and the future of drug-resistant tuberculosis. *Microb. Drug Resist.*, 2004, 10, 280-285.

[22] Telenti, A; Honore, N; Bernasconi, C; March, J; Ortega, A; Heym, B; Takiff, HE; Cole, ST. Genotypic assessment of isoniazid and rifampin resistance in *Mycobacterium tuberculosis*: A blind study at reference laboratory level. *J. Clin. Microbiol.*, 1997, 35, 719-723.

[23] Ramaswamy, S; Musser, JM. Molecular genetic basis of antimicrobial agent resistance in *Mycobacterium tuberculosis*: 1998 update. *Tuber. Lung Dis.*, 1998, 79, 3-29.

[24] Zhang, Y; Permar, S; Sun, ZH. Conditions that may affect the results of susceptibility testing of *Mycobacterium tuberculosis* to pyrazinamide. *J. Med. Microbiol.*, 2002, 51, 42-49.

[25] Zhang, Y; Wade, MM; Scorpio, A; Zhang, H; Sun, ZH. Mode of action of pyrazinamide: Disruption of *Mycobacterium tuberculosis* membrane transport and energetics by pyrazinoic acid. *J. Antimicrob. Chemother.*, 2003, 52, 790-795.

[26] Scorpio, A; Zhang, Y. Mutations in *pncA*, a gene encoding pyrazinamidase/nicotinamidase, cause resistance to the antituberculous drug pyrazinamide in tubercle bacillus. *Nat. Med.*, 1996, 2, 662-667.

[27] Scorpio, A; Lindholm-Levy, P; Heifets, L; Gilman, R; Siddiqi, S; Cynamon, M; Zhang, Y. Characterization of pncA mutations in pyrazinamide-resistant *Mycobacterium tuberculosis. Antimicrob. Agents Chemother.*, 1997, 41, 540-543.

[28] Morlock, GP; Crawford, JT; Butler, WR; Brim, SE; Sikes, D; Mazurek, GH; Woodley, CL; Cooksey, RC. Phenotypic characterization of pncA mutants of *Mycobacterium tuberculosis. Antimicrob. Agents Chemother.*, 2000, 44, 2291-2295.

[29] Telenti, A; Philipp, WJ; Sreevatsan, S; Bernasconi, C; Stockbauer, KE; Wieles, B; Musser, JM; Jacobs, WR. The emb operon, a gene cluster of *Mycobacterium tuberculosis* involved in resistance to ethambutol. *Nat. Med.*, 1997, 3, 567-570.

[30] Ramaswamy, SV; Amin, AG; Goksel, S; Stager, CE; Dou, SJ; El Sahly, H; Moghazeh, SL; Kreiswirth, BN; Musser, JM. Molecular genetic analysis of nucleotide polymorphisms associated with ethambutol resistance in human isolates of *Mycobacterium tuberculosis. Antimicrob. Agents Chemother.*, 2000, 44, 326-336.

[31] Moazed, D; Noller, HF. Interaction of antibiotics with functional sites in 16S ribosomal-RNA. *Nature*, 1987, 327, 389-394.

[32] Liu, XQ; Gillham, NW; Boynton, JE. Chloroplast ribosomal protein gene RPS12 of *Chlamydomonas reinhardtii*. Wild-type sequence,

mutation to streptomycin resistance and dependence, and function in *Escherichia coli*. *J. Biol. Chem.*, 1989, 264, 16100-16108.

[33] Gauthier, A; Turmel, M; Lemieux, C. Mapping of chloroplast mutations conferring resistance to antibiotics in *Chlamydomonas*: Evidence for a novel site of streptomycin resistance in the small subunit rRNA. *Mol. Gen. Genet.*, 1988, 214, 192-197.

[34] Drlica, K; Malik, M. Fluoroquinolones: Action and resistance. *Curr. Top. Med. Chem.*, 2003, 3, 249-282.

[35] Zhang, Y; Jacobs jr., R. Mechanism of drug action, drug resistance and drug tolerance in *Mycobacterium tuberculosis*: Expected phenotypes from evolutionary pressure from a highly successful pathogen. In: Kaufmann, HES; Rubin, E. (eds.). *Handbook of Tuberculosis: Molecular Biology and Biochemistry*, Weinhaim: Wiley-VCH; 2008; 323-378.

[36] Flynn, JL. Imunology of tuberculosis and implications in vaccine development. *Tuberculosis*, 2004, 84, 93-101.

[37] Ballell, L; Field, RA; Duncan, K; Young, RJ. New small-molecule synthetic antimycobacterials. *Antimicrob. Agents Chemother.*, 2005, 49, 2153-2163.

[38] Vinsova, J; Imramovsky, A; Jampilek, J; Monreal, JF; Dolezal, M. Recent advances on isoniazide derivatives. *Anti-Infect. Agents Med. Chem.*, 2008, 7, 1-20.

[39] Ventura, C; Martins, F. Application of quantitative structur-activity relationships to the modeling of antitubercular compounds. 1. The hydrazide family. *J. Med. Chem.*, 2008, 51, 612-624.

[40] Carvalho, SA; da Silva, EF; de Souza, MVN; Lourenco, MCS; Vicente, FR. Synthesis and antimycobacterial evaluation of new *trans*-cinnamic acid hydrazide derivatives. *Bioorg. Med. Chem. Lett.*, 2008, 18, 538-541.

[41] Imramovsky, A; Polanc, S; Vinsova, J; Kocevar, M; Jampilek, J; Reckova, Z; Kaustova, J. A new modification of anti-tubercular active molecules. *Bioorg. Med. Chem.*, 2007, 15, 2551-2559.

[42] Scior, T; Garces-Eisele, SJ. Isoniazid is not a lead compound for its pyridyl ring derivatives, isonicotinoyl amides, hydrazides, and hydrazones: A critical review. *Curr. Med. Chem.*, 2006, 13, 2205-2219.

[43] Oliveira, JS; Sousa, EHS; Basso, LA; Palaci, M; Dietze, R; Santos, DS; Moreira, IS. An inorganic iron complex that inhibits wild-type and an

isoniazid-resistant mutant 2-*trans*-enoyl-ACP (CoA) reductase from *Mycobacterium tuberculosis*. *Chem. Commun.*, 2004, 3, 312-313.

[44] Oliveira, JS; de Sousa, EHS; de Souza, ON; Moreira, IS; Santos, DS; Basso, LA. Slow-onset inhibition of 2-*trans*-enoyl-ACP (CoA) reductase from *Mycobacterium tuberculosis* by an inorganic complex. *Curr. Pharm. Design*, 2006, 12, 2409-2424.

[45] Shaharyar, M; Siddiqui, AA; Ali, MA; Sriram, D; Yogeeswari, P. Synthesis and *in vitro* antimycobacterial activity of N^1-nicotinoyl-3-(4′-hydroxy-3′-methylphenyl)-5-[(sub)phenyl]-2-pyrazolines. *Bioorg. Med. Chem. Lett.*, 2006, 16, 3947-3949.

[46] Ali, MA; Yar, MS. Synthesis and antimycobacterial activity of novel 4-[5-(substituted phenyl)-1-phenyl-4,5-dihydro-1*H*-3-pyrazolyl]-2-methylphenol derivatives. *Med. Chem. Res.*, 2007, 15, 463-470.

[47] da Silva, PEA; Ramos, DF; Bonacorso, HG; de la Iglesia, AI; Oliveira, MR; Coelho, T; Navarini, J; Morbidoni, HR; Zanatta, N; Martins, MAP. Synthesis and *in vitro* antimycobacterial activity of 3-substituted 5-hydroxy-5-trifluoro[chloro]methyl-4,5-dihydro-1*H*-1-(isonicotinoyl) pyrazoles. *Int. J. Antimicrob. Agents*, 2008, 32, 139-144.

[48] Ali, MA; Yar, MS; Kumar, M; Pandian, GS. Synthesis and antitubercular activity of substituted novel pyrazoline derivatives. *Nat. Prod. Res.*, 2007, 21, 575-579.

[49] Navarrete-Vazquez, G; Molina-Salinas, GM; Duarte-Fajardo, ZV; Vargas-Villarreal, J; Estrada-Soto, S; Gonzalez-Salazar, F; Hernandez-Nuneza, E; Said-Fernandez, S. Synthesis and antimycobacterial activity of 4-(5-substituted-1,3,4-oxadiazol-2-yl)pyridines. *Bioorg. Med. Chem.*, 2007, 15, 5502-5508.

[50] Sriram, D; Yogeeswari, P; Priya, DY. Antimycobacterial activity of novel *N*-(substituted)-2-isonicotinoylhydrazinocarbothioamide endowed with high activity towards isoniazid resistant tuberculosis. *Biomed. Pharmacother.*, 2009, 63, 36-39.

[51] Klimesova, V; Koci, J; Waisser; K; Kaustova, J; Mollmann, U. Preparation and *in vitro* evaluation of benzylsulfanyl benzoxazole derivatives as potential antituberculosis agents. *Eur. J. Med. Chem.*, 2009, 44, 2286-2293.

[52] Zhang, Y; Post-Martens, K; Denkin, S. New drug candidates and therapeutic targets for tuberculosis therapy. *Drug Discov. Today*, 2006, 11, 21-27.

[53] Rothstein, DM; Hartman, AD; Cynamon, MH; Eisenstein, BI. Development potential of rifalazil. *Expert Opin. Inv. Drugs*, 2003, 12, 255-271.

[54] Rothstein, DM; Shalish, C; Murphy, CK; Sternlicht, A; Campbell, LA. Development potential of rifalazil and other benzoxazinorifamycins. *Expert Opin. Inv. Drugs*, 2006, 15, 603-623.

[55] Hudson, A; Imamura, T; Gutteridge, W; Kanyok, T; Nunn, P. The current anti-TB drug research and development pipeline. 1st edition. Geneva: World Health Organization; 2003.

[56] Reddy, VM; Nadadhur, G; Daneluzzi, D; Dimova, V; Gangadharam, PRJ. Antimycobacterial activity of a new rifamycin derivative, 3-(4-cinnamylpiperazinyl iminomethyl) rifamycin SV (T9). *Antimicrob. Agents Chemother.*, 1995, 39, 2320-2324.

[57] Figueiredo, R; Moiteiro, C; Medeiros, MA; da Silva, PA; Ramos, D; Spies, F; Ribeiro, MO; Lourenço, MCS; Junior, IN; Gaspar, MM; Cruz, MEM, Curto, MJM; Franzblau, SG; Orozco, H; Aguilar, D; Hernandez-Pando, R; Costa, MC. Synthesis and evaluation of rifabutin analogs against *Mycobacterium avium* and $H_{37}Rv$, MDR and NRP *Mycobacterium tuberculosis*. *Bioorg. Med. Chem.*, 2009, 17, 503-511.

[58] Sriram, D; Yogeeswari, P; Reddy, SP. Synthesis of pyrazinamide Mannich bases and its antitubercular properties. *Bioorg. Med. Chem. Lett.*, 2006, 16, 2113-2116.

[59] Speirs, RJ; Welch, JT; Cynamon, MH. Activity of *n*-propyl pyrazinoate against pyrazinamide-resistant *Mycobacterium tuberculosis*: Investigations into mechanism of action of and mechanism of resistance to pyrazinamide. *Antimicrob. Agents Chemother.*, 1995, 39, 1269-1271.

[60] Cynamon, MH; Speirs, RJ; Welch, JT. *In vitro* antimycobacterial activity of 5-chloropyrazinamide. *Antimicrob. Agents Chemother.*, 1998, 42, 462-463.

[61] Dolezal, M; Cmedlova, P; Palek, L; Vinsova, J; Kunes, J; Buchta, V; Jampilek, J; Kralova, K. Synthesis and antimycobacterial evaluation of substituted pyrazinecarboxamides. *Eur. J. Med. Chem.*, 2008, 43, 1105-1113.

[62] Tewari, N; Tiwari, VK; Tripathi, RP; Chaturvedi, V; Srivastava, A; Srivastava, R; Shukla, PK; Chaturvedi, AK; Gaikwad, A; Sinha, S; Srivastava, BS. Synthesis of galactopyranosyl amino alcohols as a new class of antitubercular and antifungal agents. *Bioorg. Med. Chem. Lett.*, 2004, 14, 329-332.

[63] Tripathi, RP; Tiwari, VK; Tewari, N; Katiyar, D; Saxena, N; Sinha, S; Gaikwad, A; Srivastava, A; Chaturvedi, V; Manju, YK; Srivastava, R; Srivastava, BS. Synthesis and antitubercular activities of bis-glycosylated diamino alcohols. *Bioorg. Med. Chem.*, 2005, 13, 5668-5679.

[64] Cynamon, MH; Sklaney, M. Gatifloxacin and ethionamide as the foundation for therapy ot tuberculosis. *Antimicrob. Agents Chemother.*, 2003, 47, 2442-2444.

[65] Nuermberger, EL; Yoshimatsu, T; Tyagi, S; Williams, K; Rosenthal, I; O'Brien, RJ; Vernon, AA; Chaisson, RE; Bishai, WR; Grosset, JH. Moxifloxacin-containing regiment of reduced duration produce a stable cure in murine tuberculosis. *Am. J. Respir. Crit. Care Med.*, 2004, 170, 1131-1134.

[66] Hu, Y; Coates, AR; Mitchison, DA. Sterilizing activities of fluoroquinolones against rifampin-tolerant population of *Mycobacterium tuberculosis*. *Antimicrob. Agents Chemother.*, 2003, 47, 653-657.

[67] Nuermberger, EL; Rosenthal, I; Tyagi, S; Williams, KN; Almeida, D; Peloquin, CA; Bishai, WR; Grosset, JH. Combination chemotherapy with the nitroimidazopyran PA-824 and first-line drugs in a murine model of tuberculosis. *Antimicrob. Agents Chemother.*, 2006, 50, 2621-2625.

[68] Tortoli, E; Dionisio, D; Fabbri, C. Evaluation of moxifloxacin activity *in vitro* against *Mycobacterium tuberculosis*, including resistant and multidrug-resistant strains. *J. Chemother.*, 2004, 16, 334-336.

[69] Anderson, DL. Sitafloxacin hydrate for bacterial infections. *Drugs Today*, 2008, 44, 489-501.

[70] Lai, CC; Tan, CK; Huang, YT; Chou, CH; Hung, CC; Yang, PC; Luh, KT; Hsueh, PR. Extensively drug-resistant *Mycobacterium tuberculosis* during a trend of decreasing drug resistance from 2000 through 2006 at a medical center in Taiwan. *Clin. Infect. Dis.*, 2008, 47, E57-E63.

[71] Dinakaran, M; Senthilkumar, P; Yogeeswari, P; China, P; Nagaraja, V; Sriram, D. Novel ofloxacin derivatives: Synthesis, antimycobacterial and toxicological evaluation. *Bioorg. Med. Chem. Lett.*, 2008, 18, 1229-1236.

[72] Senthilkumar, P; Dinakaran, M; Yogeeswari, P; Sriram, D; China, A; Nagaraja, V. Synthesis and antimycobacterial activities of novel 6-nitroquinolone-3-carboxylic acids. *Eur. J. Med. Chem.*, 2009, 44, 345-358.

[73] Senthilkumar, P; Dinakaran, M; Yogeeswari, P; China, A; Nagaraja, V; Sriram, D. Antimycobacterial activities of novel fluoroquinolones. *Biomed. Pharmacother.*, 2009, 63, 27-35.

[74] Rivers, EC; Mancera, RL. New anti-tuberculosis drugs in clinical trials with novel mechanisms of action. *Drug Discov. Today*, 2008, 13, 1090-1098.

[75] Nam, HS; Koh, WJ; Kwon, OJ; Cho, SN; Shim, TS. Daily half-dose linezolid for the treatment of intractable multidrug-resistant tuberculosis. *Int. J. Antimicrob. Agents*, 2009, 33, 92-93.

[76] Prammananan, T; Chaiprasert, A; Leechawengwongs, M. *In vitro* activity of linezolid against multidrug-resistant tuberculosis (MDR-TB) and extensively drug-resistant (XDR)-TB isolates. *Int. J. Antimicrob. Agents*, 2009, 33, 190-191.

[77] Corti, G; Cinelli, R; Paradisi, F. Clinical and microbiologic efficacy and safety profile of linezolid, a new oxazolidinone antibiotic. *Int. J. Antimicrob. Agents*, 2000, 16, 527-530.

[78] Erturan, Z; Uzun, M. *In vitro* activity of linezolid against multidrug-resistant *Mycobacterium tuberculosis* isolates. *Int. J. Antimicrob. Agents*, 2005, 26, 78-80.

[79] von der Lippe, B; Sandven, P; Brubakk, O. Efficacy and safety of linezolid in multidrug resistant tuberculosis (MDR-TB) – a report of ten cases. *J. Infect.*, 2006, 52, 92-96.

[80] Park, IN; Hong, SB; Oh, YM; Kim, MN; Lim, CM; Lee, SD; Koh, Y; Kim, WS; Kim, DS; Kim, WD; Shim, TS. Efficacy and tolerability of daily-half dose linezolid in patients with intractable multidrug-resistant tuberculosis. *J. Antimicrob. Chemother.*, 2006, 58, 701-704.

[81] Fortun, J; Martin-Davila, P; Navas, E; Perez-Elias, MJ; Cobo, J; Tato, M; de la Pedrosa, EGG; Gomez-Mampaso, E; Moreno, S. Linezolid for the treatment of multidrug-resistant tuberculosis. *J. Antimicrob. Chemother.*, 2005, 56, 180-185.

[82] Swaney, SM; Aoki, H; Ganoza, MC; Shinabarger, DL. The oxazolidinone linezolid inhibits initiation of protein synthesis in bacteria. *Antimicrob. Agents Chemother.*, 1998, 42, 3251-3255.

[83] Barbachyn, MR; Hutchinson, DK; Brickner, SJ; Cynamon, MH; Kilburn, JO; Klemens, SP; Glickman, SE; Grega, KC; Hendges, SK; Toops, DS; Ford, CW; Zurenko, GE. Identification of a novel oxazolidinone (U-100480) with potent antimycobacterial activity. *J. Med. Chem.*, 1996, 39, 680-685.

[84] Cynamon, MH; Klemens, SP; Sharpe, CA; Chase, S. Activities of several novel oxazolidinones against *Mycobacterium tuberculosis* in a murine model. *Antimicrob. Agents Chemother.*, 1999, 43, 1189-1191.

[85] Vera-Cabrera, L; Castro-Garza, J; Rendon, A; Ocampo-Candiani, J; Welsh, O; Hak Choi, S; Blackwood, K; Molina-Torres, K. *In vitro* susceptibility of *Mycobacterium tuberculosis* clinical isolates to garenoxacin and DA-7867. *Antimicrob. Agents Chemother.*, 2005, 49, 4351-4353.

[86] Andries, K; Verhasselt, P; Guillemont, J; Gohlmann, HWH; Neefs, JM; Winkler, H; Van Gestel, J; Timmerman, P; Zhu, M; Lee, E; Williams, P; de Chaffoy, D; Huitric, E; Hoffner, S; Cambau, E; Truffot-Pernot, C; Lounis, N; Jarlier, V. A diarylquinoline drug active on the ATP synthase of *Mycobacterium tuberculosis*. *Science*, 2005, 307, 223-227.

[87] Huitric, E; Verhasselt, P; Andries, K; Hoffner, SE. *In vitro* antimycobacterial spectrum of a diarylquinoline ATP synthase inhibitor. *Antimicrob. Agents Chemother.*, 2007, 51, 4202-4204.

[88] Koul, A; Dendouga, N; Vergauwen, K; Molenberghs, B; Vranckx, L; Willebrords, R; Ristic, Z; Lill, H; Dorange, I; Guillemont, J; Bald, D; Andries, K. Diarylquinolines target subunit c of mycobacterial ATP synthase. *Nat. Chem. Biol.*, 2007, 3, 323-324.

[89] Lounis, N; Veziris, N; Chauffour, A; Truffot-Pernot, C; Adries, K; Jarlier, V. Combinations of R207910 with drugs used to treat multidrug-resistant tuberculosis have the potential to shorten treatment duration. *Antimicrob. Agents Chemother.*, 2006, 50, 3543-3547.

[90] Ibrahim, M; Andries, K; Lounis, N; Chauffour, A; Truffot-Pernot, C; Jarlier, V; Veziris, N. Synergistic activity of R207910 combined with pyrazinamide against murine tuberculosis. *Antimicrob. Agents Chemother.*, 2007, 51, 1011-1015.

[91] Koul, A; Vranckx, L; Dendouga, N; Balemans, W; Van den Wyngaert, I; Vergauwen, K; Goehlmann, HWH; Willebrords, R; Poncelet, A; Guillemont, J; Bald, D; Andries, K. Diarylquinolines are bactericidal for dormant mycobacteria as a result of disturbed ATP homeostasis. *J. Biol. Chem.*, 2008, 283, 25273-25280.

[92] Lenaerts, AJ; Gruppo, V; Marietta, KS; Johnson, CM; Driscoll, DK; Tompkins, NM; Rose, JD; Reynolds, RC; Orme, IM. Preclinical testing of the nitroimidazopyran PA-824 for activity against *Mycobacterium tuberculosis* in a series of *in vitro* and *in vivo* models. *Antimicrob. Agents Chemother.*, 2005, 49, 2294-2301.

[93] Stover, CK; Warrener, P; VanDevanter, DR; Sherman, DR; Arain, TM; Langhorne, MH; Anderson, SW; Towell, JA; Yuan, Y; McMurray, DN; Kreiswirth, BN; Barry, CE; Baker, WR. A small-molecule nitroimidazopyran drug candidate for the treatment of tuberculosis. *Nature*, 2000, 405, 962-966.

[94] Dubnau, E; Chan, J; Raynaud, C; Mohan, VP; Laneelle, MA; Yu, KM; Quemard, A; Smith, I; Daffe, M. Oxygenated mycolic acids are necessary for virulence of *Mycobacterium tuberculosis* in mice. *Mol. Microbiol.*, 2000, 36, 630-637.

[95] Tyagi, S; Nuermberger, E; Yoshimatsu, T; Williams, K; Rosenthal, I; Lounis, N; Bishai, W; Grosset, J. Bactericidal activity of the nitroimidazopyran PA-824 in a murine model of tuberculosis. *Antimicrob. Agents Chemother.*, 2005, 49, 2289-2293.

[96] Matsumoto, M; Hashizume, H; Tomishige, T; Kawasaki, M; Tsubouchi, H; Sasaki, H; Shimokawa, Y; Komatsu, M. OPC-67683, a nitro-dihydro-imidazooxazole derivative with promising action against tuberculosis *in vitro* and in mice. *PLoS Med.*, 2006, 3, 2131-2144.

[97] Cole, ST; Alzari, PM. Towards new tuberculosis drugs. *Biochem. Soc. Trans.*, 2007, 35, 1321-1324.

[98] Deidda, D; Lampis, G; Fioravanti, R; Biava, M; Porretta, GC; Zanetti, S; Pompei, R. Bactericidal activities of the pyrrole derivative BM212 against multidrug-resistant and intramacrophagic *Mycobacterium tuberculosis* strains. *Antimicrob. Agents Chemother.*, 1998, 42, 3035-3037.

[99] Biava, M; Porretta, GC; Poce, G; Deidda, D; Pompei, R; Tafi, A; Manetti, F. Antimycobacterial compounds. Optimization of the BM 212 structure, the lead compound for a new pyrrole derivative class. *Bioorg. Med. Chem.*, 2005, 13, 1221-1230.

[100] Biava, M; Porretta, GC; Deidda, D; Pompei, R; Tafi, A; Manetti, F. Antimycobacterial compounds. New pyrrole derivatives of BM212. *Bioorg. Med. Chem.*, 2004, 12, 1453-1458.

[101] Biava, M; Porretta, GC; Poce, G; Supino, S; Deidda, D; Pompei, R; Molicotti, P; Manetti, F; Botta, M. Antimycobacterial agents. Novel diarylpyrrole derivatives of BM212 endowed with high activity toward *Mycobacterium tuberculosis* and low cytotoxicity. *J. Med. Chem.*, 2006, 49, 4946-4952.

[102] Nikonenko, BV; Protopopova, M; Sarnala, R; Einck, L; Nacy, CA. Drug therapy of experimental tuberculosis (TB): Improved outcome by

combining SQ109, a new diamine antibiotic, with existing TB drugs. *Antimicrob. Agents Chemother.*, 2007, 51, 1563-1565.

[103] Jia, J; Tomaszewski, JE; Hanrahan, C; Coward, L; Noker, P; Gorman, G; Nikonenko, B; Protopopova, M. Pharmacodynamics and pharmacokinetics of SQ109, new diamine-based antitubercular drug. *Br. J. Pharmacol.*, 2005, 144, 80-87.

[104] Jia, L; Noker, PE; Coward, L; Gorman, GS; Protopopova, M; Tomaszewski, JE. Interspecies pharmacokinetics and *in vitro* metabolism of SQ109. *Br. J. Pharmacol.*, 2006, 147, 476-485.

[105] Protopopova, M; Hanrahan, C; Nikonenko, B; Sarnala, R; Chen, P; Gearhart, J; Einck, L; Nacy, CA. Identification of a new antitubercular drug candidate, SQ109, from combinatorial library of 1,2-ethylenediamines. *J. Antimicrob. Chemother.*, 2005, 56, 968-974.

[106] Chen, P; Gearhart, J; Protopopova, M; Einck, L; Nacy, CA. Synergistic interactions of SQ109, a new ethylene diamine, with front-line antitubercular drugs *in vitro*. *J. Antimicrob. Chemother.*, 2006, 58, 332-337.

[107] LL-3858. *Tuberculosis*, 2008, 88, 126.

[108] Hampton, T. TB drug research picks up the pace. *JAMA*, 2005, 293, 2705-2707.

[109] Tomioka, H; Tatano, Y; Yasumoto, K; Shimizu, T. Recent advances in antituberculous drug development and novel drug targets. *Expert Rev. Resp. Med.*, 2008, 2, 455-471.

[110] Cole, ST; Brosch, R; Parkhill, J; Garnier, T; Churcher, C; Harris, D; Gordon, SV; Eiglmeier, K; Gas, S; Barry, CE; Tekaia, F; Badcock, K; Basham, D; Brown, D; Chillingworth, T; Connor, R; Davies, R; Devlin, K; Feltwell, T; Gentles, S; Hamlin, N; Holroyd, S; Hornby, T; Jagels, K; Krogh, A; McLean, J; Moule, S; Murphy, L; Oliver, K; Osborne, J; Quail, MA; Rajandream, MA; Rogers, J; Rutter, S; Seeger, K; Skelton, J; Squares, R; Squares, S; Sulston, JE; Taylor, K; Whitehead, S; Barrell, BG. Deciphering the biology of *Mycobacterium tuberculosis* from the complete genome sequence. *Nature*, 1998, 393, 537-544.

[111] Hong, X; Hopfinger, AJ. Molecular modeling and simulation of *Mycobacterium tuberculosis* cell wall permeability. *Biomacromolecules*, 2004, 5, 1066-1077.

[112] Brennan, PJ; Nikaido, H. The envelope of mycobacteria. *Annu. Rev. Biochem.*, 1995, 64, 29-63.

[113] http://www.ncbi.nlm.nih.gov/bookshelf/br.fcgi?book=glyco2&part=ch2 0&rendertype=figure&id=ch20.f8

[114] van Rensburg, CEJ; Joone, GK; Siegel, FA; Matlola, NM; O'Sullivan, JF. *In vitro* investigation of the antimicrobial activities of a novel tetramethylpiperidine-substituted phenazines against *Mycobacterium tubeculosis*. *Chemotherapy*, 2000, 46, 43-48.

[115] Reddy, VM; O'Sullivan, JF; Gangadharam, PRJ. Antimycobacterial activities of riminophenazines. *J. Antimicrob. Chemother.*, 1999, 43, 615-623.

[116] Matsumoto, M; Hashizume, H; Tsubouchi, H; Sasaki, H; Itotani, M; Kuroda, H; Tomishige, T; Kawasaki, M; Komatsu, M. Screening for novel antituberculosis agents that are effective against multidrug resistant tuberculosis. *Curr. Top. Med. Chem.*, 2007, 7, 499-507.

[117] Reddy, VM; Nadadhur, G; Daneluzzi, D; O'Sullivan, JF; Gangadharam, PRJ. Antituberculosis activities of clofazimine and its new analogs B4154 and B4157. *Antimicrob. Agents Chemother.*, 1996, 633-636.

[118] Schroeder, EK; de Souza, ON; Santos, DS; Blanchard, JS; Basso, LA. Drugs that inhibit mycolic acid biosynthesis in *Mycobacterium tuberculosis*. *Curr. Pharm. Biotechnol.*, 2002, 3, 197-225.

[119] Barry, PJ; O'Connor, TM. Novel agents in the management of *Mycobacterium tuberculosis* disease. *Curr. Med. Chem.*, 2007, 14, 2000-2008.

[120] Parrish, NM; Kuhajda, FP; Heine, HS; Bishai, WR; Dick, JD. Antimycobacterial activity of cerulenin and its effects on lipid biosynthesis. *J. Antimicrob. Chemother.*, 1999, 43, 219-26.

[121] Chang, Y; Fox, BG. Identification of Rv3230c as the NADPH oxidoreductase of a two-protein DesA3 acyl-CoA desaturase in *Mycobacterium tuberculosis* $H_{37}Rv$. *Biochemistry*, 2006, 45, 13476-13486.

[122] Chang, Y; Wesenberg, GE; Bingman, CA; Fox, BG. *In vivo* inactivation of the mycobacterial integral membrane stearoyl coenzyme a desaturase DesA3 by a C-terminus-specific degradation process. *J. Bacteriol.*, 2008, 190, 6686-6696.

[123] Kordulakova, J; Janin, YL; Liav, A; Barilone, N; Dos Vultos, T; Rauzier, J; Brennan, PJ; Gicquel, B; Jackson, M. Isoxyl activation is required for bacteriostatic activity against *Mycobacterium tuberculosis*. *Antimicrob. Agents Chemother.*, 2007, 51, 3824-3829.

[124] Phetsuksiri, B; Jackson, M; Scherman, H; McNeil, M; Besra, GS; Baulard, AR; Slayden, RA; DeBarber, AE; Barry, CE; Baird, MS; Crick, DC; Brennan, PJ. Unique mechanism of action of the thiourea drug isoxyl on *Mycobacterium tuberculosis*. *J. Biol. Chem.*, 2003, 278, 53123-53130.

[125] DeBarber, AE; Mdluli, K; Bosman, N; Bekker, LG; Barry, CE. Ethionamide activation and sensitivity in multidrug-resistant *Mycobacterium tuberculosis*. *Proc. Natl. Acad. Sci. U.S.A.*, 2000, 97, 9677-9682.

[126] Phetsuksiri, B; Baulard, AR; Cooper, AR; Minnikin, DE; Douglas, JD; Besra, GS; Brennan, PJ. Antimycobacterial activities of isoxyl and new derivatives through the inhibition of mycolic acid synthesis. *Antimicrob. Agents Chemother.*, 1999, 43, 1042-1051.

[127] Sriram, D; Yogeeswari, P; Dinakaran, M; Thirumurugan, R. Antimycobacterial activity of novel 1-(5-cyclobutyl-1,3-oxazol-2-yl)-3-(sub)phenyl/pyridylthiourea compounds endowed with high activity toward multidrug-resistant *Mycobacterium tuberculosis*. *J. Antimicrob. Chemother.*, 2007, 59, 1194-1196.

[128] Hackbarth, CJ; Chen, DZ; Lewis, JG; Clark, K; Mangold, JB; Cramer, JA; Margolis, PS; Wang, W; Koehn, J; Wu, C; Lopez, S; Withers, GIII; Gu, H; Dunn, E; Kulathila, R; Pan, SH; Porter, WL; Jacobs, J; Trias, J; Patel, DV; Weidmann, B; White, RJ; Yuan, Z. *N*-Alkyl urea hydroxamic acids as a new class of peptide deformylase inhibitors with antibacterial activity. *Antimicrob. Agents Chemother.*, 2002, 46, 2752-2764.

[129] Teo, JWP; Thayalan, P; Beer, D; Yap, ASL; Nanjundappa, M; Ngew, X; Duraiswamy, J; Liung, S; Dartois, V; Schreiber, M; Hasan, S; Cynamon, M; Ryder, NS; Yang, X; Weidmann, B; Bracken, K; Dick, T; Mukherjee, K. Peptide deformylase inhibitors as potent antimycobacterial agents. *Antimicrob. Agents Chemother.*, 2006, 50, 3665-3673.

[130] Pichota, A; Duraiswamy, J; Yin, Z; Keller, TH; Alam, J; Liung, S; Lee, G; Ding, M; Wang, G; Chan, WL; Schreiber, M; Maa, I; Beer, D; Ngew, X; Mukherjee, K; Nanjundappa, M; Teo, JWP; Thayalan, P; Yap, A; Dick, T; Meng, W; Xu, M; Koehn, J; Pan, SH; Clark, K; Xie, X; Shoen, C; Cynamon, M. Peptide deformylase inhibitors of *Mycobacterium tuberculosis*: Synthesis, structural investigations, and biological results. *Bioorg. Med. Chem. Lett.*, 2008, 18, 6568-6572.

[131] He, X; Alian, A; Stroud, R; de Montellano, PRO. Pyrrolidine carboxamides as a novel class of inhibitors of enoyl acyl carrier protein reductase from *Mycobacterium tuberculosis*. *J. Med. Chem.*, 2006, 49, 6308-6323.

[132] Hea, X; Alian, A; de Montellano, PRO. Inhibition of the *Mycobacterium tuberculosis* enoyl acyl carrier protein reductase InhA by arylamides. *Bioorg. Med. Chem.*, 2007, 15, 6649-6658.

[133] McMurry, LM; Oethinger, M; Levy, SB. Triclosan targets lipid synthesis. *Nature*, 1998, 394, 531-532.

[134] Sullivan, TJ; Truglio, JJ; Boyne, ME; Novichenok, P; Zhang, X; Stratton, CF; Li, HJ; Kaur, T; Amin, SA; Johnson, F; Slayden, RA; Kisker, C; Tonge, PJ. High affinity InhA inhibitors with activity against drug-resistant strains of *Mycobacterium tuberculosis*. *ACS Chem. Biol.*, 2006, 1, 43-53.

[135] Andrade, CH; Pasqualoto, KFM; Zaim, MH; Ferreira, EI. Rational approach in the new antituberculosis agent design: Inhibitors of InhA, the enoyl-ACP reductase from *Mycobacterium tuberculosis*. *Rev. Bras. Cienc. Farm.*, 2008, 44, 167-179.

[136] Lu, H; Tonge, PJ. Inhibitors of FabI, an enzyme drug target in the bacterial fatty acid biosynthesis pathway. *Acc. Chem. Res.*, 2008, 41, 11-20.

[137] Lowary, TL. Recent progress towards the identification of inhibitors of mycobacterial cell wall polysaccharide biosynthesis. *Mini Rev. Med. Chem.*, 2003, 3, 689-702.

[138] Naresh, K; Bharati, BK; Jayaraman, N; Chatterji, D. Synthesis and mycobacterial growth inhibition activities of bivalent and monovalent arabinofuranoside containing alkyl glycosides. *Org. Biomol. Chem.*, 2008, 6, 2388-2393.

[139] Subramaniam, V; Gurcha, SS; Besra, GS; Lotary, TL. Modified mannose disaccharides as substrates and inhibitors of a polyprenol monophosphomannose-dependent alpha-($1\rightarrow6$)-mannosyltransferase involved in mycobacterial lipoarabinomannan biosynthesis. *Bioorg. Med. Chem.*, 2005, 13, 1083-1094.

[140] Eoh, H; Brennan, PJ; Crick, DC. The *Mycobacterium tuberculosis* MEP (2C-methyl-D-erythritol 4-phosphate) pathway as a new drug target. *Tuberculosis*, 2009, 89, 1-11.

[141] Eoh, H; Brown, AC; Buetow, L; Hunter, WN; Parish, T; Kaur, D; Brennan, PJ; Crick, DC. Characterization of the *Mycobacterium*

tuberculosis 4-diphosphocytidyl-2-C-methyl-D-erythritol synthase: Potential for drug development. *J. Bacteriol.*, 2007, 189, 8922-8927.

[142] Parrish, NM; Ko, CG; Hughes, MA; Townsed, CA; Dick, JD. Effect of *n*-octanesulphonylacetamide (OSA) on ATP and protein expression in *Mycobacterium bovis* BCG. *J. Antimicrob. Chemother., 2004, 54, 722-729.

[143] Koga, T; Fukuoka, T; Doi, N; Harasaki, T; Inoue, H; Hotoda, H; Kakuta, M; Muramatsu, Y; Yamamura, N; Hoshi, M; Hirota T. Activity of capuramycin analogues against *Mycobacterium tuberculosis*, *Mycobacterium avium* and *Mycobacterium intracellulare in vitro* and *in vivo*. *J. Antimicrob. Chemother.*, 2004, 54, 755-760.

[144] Tangallapally, RP; Yendapally, R; Daniels, AJ; Lee, REB; Lee, RE. Nitrofurans as novel anti-tuberculosis agents: Identification, development and evaluation. *Curr. Top. Med. Chem.*, 2007, 7, 509-526.

[145] Tangallapally, RP; Yendapally, R; Lee, REB; Lenaerts, AJM; Lee, RE. Synthesis and evaluation of cyclic secondary amine substituted phenyl and benzyl nitrofuranyl amides as novel antituberculosis agents. *J. Med. Chem.*, 2005, 48, 8261-8269.

[146] Tangallapally, RP; Lee, REB; Lenaerts, AJM; Lee, RE. Synthesis of a new and potent analogues of anti-tuberculosis agent 5-nitro-furan-2-carboxylic acid 4-(4-benzyl-piperazin-1-yl)-benzylamide with improved bioavailability. *Bioorg. Med. Chem. Lett.*, 2006, 16, 2584-2589.

[147] Tangallapally, RP; Sun, D; Rakesh; Budha, N; Lee, REB; Lenaerts, AJM; Meibohma, B; Lee, RE. Discovery of novel isoxazolines as anti-tuberculosis agents. *Bioorg. Med. Chem. Lett.*, 2007, 17, 6638-6642.

[148] Liu, J; Ren, HP. Tuberculosis: Current treatment and new drug development. *Anti-Infect. Agents Med. Chem.*, 2006, 5, 331-344.

[149] Ghannoum, MA; Rice, LB. Antifungal agents: Mode of action, mechanisms of resistance, and correlation of these mechanisms with bacterial resistance. *Clin. Microbiol. Rev.*, 1999, 12, 501-517.

[150] McLean, KJ; Dunford, AJ; Neeli, R; Driscoll, MD; Munro, AW. Structure, function and drug targeting in *Mycobacterium tuberculosis* cytochrome P450 systems. *Arch. Biochem. Biophys.*, 2007, 464, 228-240.

[151] Mamolo, MG; Zampieri, D; Vio, L; Fermeglia, M; Ferrone, M; Pricl, S; Scialino, G; Banfi, E. Antimycobacterial activity of new 3-substituted 5-(pyridin-4-yl)-3*H*-1,3,4-oxadiazol-2-one and 2-thione derivatives.

Preliminary molecular modeling investigations. *Bioorg. Med. Chem.*, 2005, 13, 3797-3809.

[152] McLean, KJ; Clift, D; Lewis, DG; Sabri, M; Balding, PR; Sutcliffe, MJ; Leys, D; Munro. AW. The preponderance of P450s in the *Mycobacterium tuberculosis* genome. *Trends Microbiol.*, 2006, 14, 220-228.

[153] Munoz-Elias, EJ; McKinney, JD. *Mycobacterium tuberculosis* isocitrate lyases 1 and 2 are jointly required for *in vivo* growth and virulence. *Nat. Med.*, 2005, 11, 638-644.

[154] Munoz-Elias, EJ; Upton, AM; Cherian, J; McKinney, JD. Role of the methylcitrate cycle in *Mycobacterium tuberculosis* metabolism, intracellular growth, and virulence. *Mol. Microbiol.*, 2006, 60, 1109-1122.

[155] Sharma, V; Sharma, S; Bentrup, KHZ; McKinney, JD; Russell, DG; Jacobs, WR; Sacchettini, JC. Structure of isocitrate lyase, a persistence factor of *Mycobacterium tuberculosis*. *Nat. Struct. Biol.*, 2000, 7, 663-668.

[156] Schloss, JV; Cleland, WW. Inhibition of isocitrate lyase by 3-nitropropionate, a reaction-intermediate analogue. *Biochemistry*, 1982, 21, 4420-4427.

[157] Tripathi, RP; Tewari, N; Dwivedi, N; Tiwari, VK. Fighting tuberculosis: An old disease with new challenges. *Med. Res. Rev.*, 2005, 25, 93-131.

[158] Li, JM; Li, N; Zhu, DY; Wan, LG; He, YL; Yang, C. Isocitrate lyase from *Mycobacterium tuberculosis* promotes survival of *Mycobacterium smegmatis* within macrophage by suppressing cell apoptosis. *Chin. Med. J.*, 2008, 121, 1114-1119.

[159] Bi, E; Lutkenhaus, J. FtsZ ring structure associated with division in *Escherichia coli*. *Nature*, 1991, 354, 161-164.

[160] Huang, Q; Tonge, PJ; Slayden, RA; Kirikae, T; Ojima, I. FtsZ: A novel target for tuberculosis drug discovery. *Curr. Top. Med. Chem.*, 2007, 7, 527-543.

[161] Ojima, I; Borella, CP; Wu, XY; Bounaud, PY; Oderda, CF; Sturm, M; Miller, ML; Chakravarty, S; Chen, J; Huang, Q; Pera, P; Brooks, TA; Baer, MR; Bernacki, RJ. Design, synthesis and structure-activity relationships of novel taxane-based multidrug resistance reversal agents. *J. Med. Chem.*, 2005, 48, 2218-2228.

[162] Huang, Q; Kirikae, T; Pepe, A; Amin, A; Respicio, L; Slayden, RA; Tonge, PJ; Ojima, I. Targeting FtsZ for antituberculosis drug discovery:

Noncytotoxic taxanes as novel antituberculosis agents. *J. Med. Chem.*, 2006, 49, 463-466.

[163] White, EL; Suling, WJ; Ross, LJ; Seitz, LE; Reynolds, RC. 2-Alkoxycarbonylaminopyridines: Inhibitors of *Mycobacterium tuberculosis* FtsZ. *J. Antimicrob. Chemother.*, 2002, 50, 111-114.

[164] Av-Gay, Y; Everett, M. The eukaryotic-like Ser/Thr protein kinases of *Mycobacterium tuberculosis. Trends Microbiol.*, 2000, 8, 238-244.

[165] Walburger, A; Koul, A; Ferrari, G; Nguyen, L; Prescianotto-Baschong, C; Huygen, K; Klebl, B; Thompson, C; Bacher, G; Pieters, J. Protein kinase G from pathogenic mycobacteria promotes survival within macrophages. *Science*, 2004, 304, 1800-1804.

[166] Szekely, R; Waczek, F; Szabadkai, I; Nemeth, G; Hegymegi-Barakonyi, B; Eros, D; Szokol, B; Pato, J; Hafenbradl, D; Satchell, J; Saint-Joanis, B; Cole, ST; Orfi, L; Klebl, BM; Keri, G. A novel drug discovery concept for tuberculosis: Inhibition of bacterial and host cell signalling. *Immunol. Lett.*, 2008, 116, 225-231.

[167] Dinakaran, M; Senthilkumar, P; Yogeeswari, P; Sriram, D. Antitubercular activities of novel benzothiazolo naphthyridone carboxylic acid derivatives endowed with high activity toward multi-drug resistant tuberculosis. *Biomed. Pharmacother.*, 2009, 63, 11-18.

[168] Dinakaran, M; Senthilkumar, P; Yogeeswari, P; China, A; Nagaraja, V; Sriram, D. Antimycobacterial activities of novel 2-(sub)-3-fluoro/nitro-5,12-dihydro-5-oxobenzothiazolo[3,2-a]quinoline-6-carboxylic acid. *Bioorg. Med. Chem.*, 2008, 16, 3408-3418.

[169] Murugesan, D; Palaniappan, S; Perumal, Y; Arnab, C; Valakunja, N; Sriram, D. Antimycobacterial and phototoxic evaluation of novel 6-fluoro/nitro-4-oxo-7-(sub)-4*H*-[1,3]thiazeto[3,2-a]quinoline-3-carboxylic acid. *Int. J. Antimicrob. Agents*, 2008, 31, 337-344.

[170] Martins, M; Viveiros, M; Ramos, J; Couto, I; Molnar, J; Boeree, M; Amaral, L. SILA 421, an inhibitor of efflux pumps of cancer cells, enhances the killing of intracellular extensively drug-resistant tuberculosis (XDR-TB). *Int. J. Antimicrob. Agents*, 2009, 33, 479-482.

[171] Amaral, L; Martins, M; Viveiros, M. Enhanced killing of intracellular multidrug-resistant *Mycobacterium tuberculosis* by compounds that affect the activity of efflux pumps. *J. Antimicrob. Chemother.*, 2007, 59, 1237-1246.

[172] de Mendonqa, JD; Ely, F; Palma, MS; Frazzon, J; Basso, LA; Santos, DS. Functional characterization by genetic complementation of *aroB*-

encoded dehydroquinate synthase from *Mycobacterium tuberculosis* $H_{37}Rv$ and its heterologous expression and purification. *J. Bacteriol.*, 2007, 189, 6246-6252.

[173] Segura-Cabrera, A; Rodriguez-Perez, MA. Structure-based prediction of Mycobacterium tuberculosis shikimate kinase inhibitors by high-throughput virtual screening. *Bioorg. Med. Chem. Lett.*, 2008, 18, 3152-3157.

[174] Gupte, A; Boshoff, HI; Wilson, DJ; Neres, J; Labello, BP; Somu, RV; Xing, C; Barry, CE; Aldrich, CC. Inhibition of siderophore biosynthesis by 2-triazole substituted analogues of 5'-O-[N-(salicyl)sulfamoyl]adenosine: Antibacterial nucleosides effective against *Mycobacterium tuberculosis*. *J. Med. Chem.*, 2008, 51, 7495-7507.

[175] Mann, S; Ploux, O. 7,8-Diaminoperlargonic acid aminotransferase from *Mycobacterium tuberculosis*, a potential therapeutic target. *FEBS J.*, 2006, 273, 4778-4789.

[176] Nathan, C; Gold, B; Lin, G; Stegman, M; de Carvalho, LPS; Vandal, O; Venugopal, A; Bryk, R. A philosophy of anti-infectives as a guide in the search for new drugs for tuberculosis. *Tuberculosis*, 2008, 88, S25-S33.

[177] Ma, YF; Stern, RJ; Scherman, MS; Vissa, VD; Yan, WX; Jones, VC; Zhang, FQ; Franzblau, SG; Lewis, WH; McNeil, MR. Drug targeting *Mycobacterium tuberculosis* cell wall synthesis: Genetics of dTDP-rhamnose synthetic enzymes and development of a microtiter plate-based screen for inhibitors of conversion of dTDP-glucose to dTDP-rhamnose. *Antimicrob. Agents Chemother.*, 2001, 45, 1407-1416.

[178] Babaoglu, K; Page, MA; Jones, VC; McNeil, MR; Dong, CJ; Naismith, JH; Lee, RE. Novel inhibitors of an emerging target in *Mycobacterium tuberculosis*; Substituted thiazolidinones as inhibitors of dTDP-rhamnose synthesis. *Bioorg. Med. Chem. Lett.*, 2003, 13, 3227-3230.

[179] Chambers, HF; Turner, J; Schecter, GF; Kawamura, M; Hopewell, PC. Imipenem for treatment of tuberculosis in mice and humans. *Antimicrob. Agents Chemother.*, 2005, 49, 2816-2821.

[180] Rastogi, N; Goh, KS; Berchel, M; Bryskier, A. *In vitro* activities of the ketolides telithromycin (HMR 3647) and HMR 3004 compared to those of clarithromycin against slowly growing mycobacteria at pHs 6.8 and 7.4. *Antimicrob. Agents Chemother.*, 2000, 44, 2848-2852.

[181] Falzari, K; Zhu, Z; Pan, D; Liu, H; Hongmanee, P; Franzblau, SG. *In vitro* and *in vivo* activities of macrolide derivatives against

Mycobacterium tuberculosis. Antimicrob. Agents Chemother., 2005, 49, 1447-1454.

[182] Dutta, NK; Mazumdarb, K; Dastidar, SG; Park, JH. Activity of diclofenac used alone and in combination with streptomycin against *Mycobacterium tuberculosis* in mice. *Int. J. Antimicrob Agents*, 2007, 30, 336-340.

[183] Dutta, NK; Mazumdar, K; Dastigar, SG; Chakrabarty, AN; Shirataki, Y; Motohashi. N. *In vitro* and *in vivo* antimycobacterial activity of an antihypertensive agent methyl-L-DOPA. *In Vivo*, 2005, 19, 539-545.

[184] Amaral, L; Kristiansen, JE; Abebe, LS; Millett, W. Inhibition of the respiration of multi-drug resistant clinical isolates of *Mycobacterium tuberculosis* by thioridazine: Potential use for initial therapy of freshly diagnosed tuberculosis. *J. Antimicrob. Chemother.*, 1996, 38, 1049-1053.

[185] Amaral, L; Kristiansen, JE; Viveiros, M; Atouguia, J. Activity of phenothiazines against antibiotic-resistant *Mycobacterium tuberculosis*: A review supporting further studies that may elucidate the potential use of thioridazine as anti-tuberculosis therapy. *J. Antimicrob. Chemother.*, 2001, 47, 505-511.

[186] Bettencourt, MV; Bosne-David, S; Amaral, L. Comparative *in vitro* activity of phenothiazines against multidrug-resistant *Mycobacterium tuberculosis*. *Int. J. Antimicrob. Agents*, 2000, 16, 69-71.

[187] Amaral, L; Martins, M; Viveiros, M; Molnar, J; Kristiansen, JE. Promising therapy of XDR-TB/MDR-TB with thioridazine an inhibitor of bacterial efflux pumps. *Curr. Drug Targets*, 2008, 9, 816-819.

[188] Thanacoody, HKR. Thioridazine: Resurrection as an antimicrobial agent? *Br. J. Clin. Pharmacol.*, 2007, 64, 566-574.

[189] Weinstein, EA; Yano, T; Li, LS; Avarbock, D; Avarbock, A; Helm, D; McColm, AA; Duncan, K; Lonsdale, JT; Rubin, H. Inhibitors of type II NADH: menaquinone oxidoreductase represent a class of antitubercular drugs. *Proc. Natl. Acad. Sci. U.S.A.*, 2005, 102, 4548-4553.

[190] Madrid, PB; Polgar, WE; Tolla, L; Tanga, MJ. Synthesis and antitubercular activity of phenothiazines with reduced binding to dopamine and serotonin receptors. *Bioorg. Med. Chem. Lett.*, 2007, 17, 3014-3017.

[191] Viveiros, M; Amaral, L. Enhancement of antibiotic activity against poly-drug resistant *Mycobacterium tuberculosis* by phenothiazine. *Int. J. Antimicrob. Agents*, 2001, 17, 225-228.

[192] Bate, AB; Kalin, JH; Fooksman, EM; Amorose, EL; Price, CM; Williams, HM; Rodig, MJ; Mitchell, MO; Cho, SH; Wang, Y; Franzblau, SG. Synthesis and antitubercular activity of quaternized promazine and promethazine derivatives. *Bioorg. Med. Chem. Lett.*, 2007, 17, 1346-1348.

[193] Martins, M; Schelz, Z; Martins, A; Molnar, J; Hajos, G; Riedl, Z; Viveiros, M; Yalcin, I; Aki-Sener, E; Amaral, L. *In vitro* and *ex vivo* activity of thioridazine derivatives against *Mycobacterium tuberculosis*. *Int. J. Antimicrob. Agents*, 2007, 29, 338-340.

[194] Grange, JM; Snell, NJC. Activity of bromhexine and ambroxol, semi-synthetic derivatives of vasicine from the Indian shrub *Adhatoda vasica*, against *Mycobacterium tuberculosis in vitro*. *J. Ethnopharmacol.*, 1996, 50, 49-53.

[195] Pathak, AK; Pathak, V; Seitz, LE; Suling, WJ; Reynold, RC. Antimycobacterial agents. 1. Thio analogues of purine. *J. Med. Chem.*, 2004, 47, 273-276.

[196] Barrow, EW; Westbrook, L; Bansal, N; Suling, WJ; Maddry, JA; Parker, WB; Barrow, WW. Antimycobacterial activity of 2-methyl-adenosine. *J. Antimicrob. Chemother.*, 2003, 52, 801-808.

[197] Kamal, A; Reddy, KS; Ahmed, SK; Khan, MNA; Sinha, RK; Yadava, JS; Arorab, SK. Anti-tubercular agents. Part 3. Benzothiadiazine as a novel scaffold for anti-*Mycobacterium* activity. *Bioorg. Med. Chem.*, 2006, 14, 650-658.

[198] Kamal, A; Ahmed, SK; Reddy, KS; Khan, MNA; Shettya, AVCRNC; Siddardha, B; Murthy, USN; Khan, IA; Kumar, M; Sharma, S; Ram, AB. Anti-tubercular agents. Part IV: Synthesis and antimycobacterial evaluation of nitroheterocyclic-based 1,2,4-benzothiadiazine. *Bioorg. Med. Chem. Lett.*, 2007, 17, 5419-5422.

[199] Kumar, RR; Perumal, S; Senthilkumar, P; Yogeeswari, P; Sriram, D. An atom efficient, solvent-free, green synthesis and antimycobacterial evaluation of 2-amino-6-methyl-4-aryl-8-[(*E*)-arylmethylidene]-5,6,7,8-tetrahydro-4*H*-pyrano[3,2-c]pyridine-3-carbonitriles. *Bioorg. Med. Chem. Lett.*, 2007, 17, 6459-6462.

[200] Villar, R; Vicente, E; Solano, B; Perez-Silanes, S; Aldana, I; Maddry, JA; Lenaerts, AJ; Franzblau, SG; Cho, SH; Monge, A; Goldman, RC. *In vitro* and *in vivo* antimycobacterial activities of ketone and amide derivatives of quinoxaline 1,4-di-*N*-oxide. *J. Antimicrob. Chemother.*, 2008, 62, 547-554.

[201] Vicente, E; Villar, R; Burguete, A; Solano, B; Perez-Silanes, S; Aldana, I; Maddry, JA; Lenaerts, AJ; Franzblau, SG; Cho, SH; Monge, A; Goldman, RC. Efficacy of quinoxaline 2-carboxylate 1,4-di-*N*-oxide derivatives in experimetnal tuberculosis. *Antimicrob. Agents Chemother.*, 2008, 52, 3321-3326.

[202] Jaso, A; Zarranz, B; Aldana, I; Monge, A. Synthesis of new quinoxaline-2-carboxylate 1,4-dioxide derivatives as anti-*Mycobacterium tuberculosis* agents. *J. Med. Chem.*, 2005, 48, 2019-2025.

[203] Kumar, RR; Perumal, S; Senthilkumar, P; Yogeeswari, P; Sriram, D. A highly atom economic, chemo-, regio- and stereoselective synthesis, and discovery of spiro-pyrido-pyrrolizines and pyrrolidines as antimycobacterial agents. *Tetrahedron*, 2008, 64, 2962-2971.

[204] Kumar, RR; Perumal, S; Senthilkumar, P; Yogeeswari, P; Sriram, D. Discovery of antimycobacterial spiro-piperidin-4-ones: An atom economic, stereoselective synthesis, and biological intervention. *J. Med. Chem.*, 2008, 51, 5731-5735.

[205] Tripathi, RP; Saxena, N; Tiwari, VK; Verma, SS; Chaturvedi, V; Manju, YK; Srivastva, AK; Gaikwad, A; Sinha, S. Synthesis and antitubercular activity of substituted phenylmethyl- and pyridylmethyl amines. *Bioorg. Med. Chem.*, 2006, 14, 8186-8196.

[206] Dwivedi, N; Tewari, N; Tiwari, VK; Chaturvedi, V; Manju, YK; Srivastava, A; Giakwad, A; Sinha, S; Tripathi, RP. An efficient synthesis of aryloxyphenyl cyclopropyl methanones: A new class of anti-mycobacterial agents. *Bioorg. Med. Chem. Lett.*, 2005, 15, 4526-4530.

[207] Katiyar, D; Tiwari, VK; Tripathi, RP; Srivastava, A; Chaturvedi, V; Srivastava, R; Srivastava, BS. Synthesis and antimycobacterial activity of 3,5-disubstituted thiadiazine thiones. *Bioorg. Med. Chem.*, 2003, 11, 4369-4375.

[208] Encarnacion-Dimayuga, R; Ramírez, MR; Luna-Herrera, J. Aerothionin, a bromotyrosine derivative with antimycobacterial activity from the marine sponge *Aplysina gerardogreeni* (Demospongia). *Pharm. Biol.*, 2003, 41, 384-387.

[209] van Klink, JW; Larsen, L; Perry, NB; Weavers, RT; Cook, GM; Bremer, PJ; MacKenzie, AD; Kirikae, T. Triketones active against antibiotic-resistant bacteria: Synthesis, structure-activity relationships, and mode of action. *Bioorg. Med. Chem.*, 2005, 13, 6651-6662.

[210] Lall, N; Meyer, JJM; Wang, Y; Bapela, NB; van Rensburg, CEJ; Fourie, B; Franzblau, SG. Characterization of intracellular activity of antitubercular constituents the roots of *Euclea natalensis*. *Pharm. Biol.*, 2005, 43, 353-357.

[211] Lall, N; Meyer, JJM. Inhibition of drug-sensitive and drug-resistant strains of *Mycobacterium tuberculosis* by diospyrin, isolated from *Euclea natalensis*. *J. Ethnopharmacol.*, 2001, 78, 213-216.

[212] Bapela, NB; Lall, N; Fourie, PB; Franzblau, SG; van Rensburg, CEJ. Activity of 7-methyljuglone in combination with antituberculous drugs against *Mycobacterium tuberculosis*. *Phytomedicine*, 2006, 13, 630-635.

[213] Mahapatra, A; Mativandlela, SPN; Binneman, B; Fourie, PB; Hamilton, CJ; Meyer, JJM; van der Kooy, F; Houghton, P; Lall, N. Activity of 7-methyljuglone derivatives against *Mycobacterium tuberculosis* and as subversive substrates for mycothiol disulfide reductase. *Bioorg. Med. Chem.*, 2007, 15, 7638-7646.

[214] Newton, SM; Lau, C; Wright, CW. A review of antimycobacterial natural products. *Phytother. Res.*, 14, 2000, 303-322.

[215] Molina-Salinas, GM; Ramos-Guerra, MC; Vargas-Villarreal, J; Mata-Cardenas, BD; Becerril-Montes, P; Said-Fernandez, S. Bactericidal activity of organic extracts from *Flourensia cernua* DC against strains of *Mycobacterium tuberculosis*. *Arch. Med. Res.*, 2006, 37, 45-49.

[216] Rojas, R; Caviedes, L; Aponte, JC; Vaisberg, AJ; Lewis, WH; Lamas, G; Sarasara, C; Gilman, RH; Hammond, GB. Aegicerin, the first oleanane triterpene with wide-ranging antimycobacterial activity, isolated from *Clavija procera*. *J. Nat. Prod.*, 2006, 69, 845-846.

[217] Camacho-Corona, MD; Ramirez-Cabrera, MA; Gonzalez-Santiago, O; Garza-Gonzalez, E; Palacios, ID; Luna-Herrera, J. Activity against drug resistant-tuberculosis strains of plants used in Mexican traditional medicine to treat tuberculosis and other respiratory diseases. *Phytother. Res.*, 2008, 22, 82-85.

[218] McGaw, LJ; Lall, N; Meyer, JJM; Eloff, JN. The potential of South African plants against *Mycobacterium* infections. *J. Ethnopharmacol.*, 2008, 119, 482-500.

INDEX

U

V

W

T